Diverticulitis Cookbook

Andrea Allison

© Copyright 2022 - All rights reserved

The content contained within this book may not be reproduced, duplicated or transmitted without direct written permission from the author or the publisher.
Under no circumstances will any blame or legal responsibility be held against the publisher, or author, for any damages, reparation, or monetary loss due to the information contained within this book. Either directly or indirectly.

Legal Notice:
This book is copyright protected. This book is only for personal use. You cannot amend, distribute, sell, use, quote or paraphrase any part, or the content within this book, without the consent of the author or publisher.

Disclaimer Notice:
Please note the information contained within this document is for educational and entertainment purposes only. All effort has been executed to present accurate, up to date, and reliable, complete information. No warranties of any kind are declared or implied. Readers acknowledge that the author is not engaging in the rendering of legal, financial, medical or professional advice. The content within this book has been derived from various sources. Please consult a licensed professional before attempting any techniques outlined in this book. By reading this document, the reader agrees that under no circumstances is the author responsible for any losses, direct or indirect, which are incurred as a result of the use of information contained within this document, including, but not limited to, — errors, omissions, or inaccuracies.

Table of Contents

Introduction	7
Chapter 1. What Is Diverticulitis?	9
Causes of Diverticulitis	10
Symptoms of Diverticulitis	11
Risk Factor	12
Diverticulitis Associated Complications	13
An Abscess	13
Perforation	13
Bleeding in the Rectal Area	13
Fistula	14
Obstruction of the Intestines	14
Options for Diverticulitis Treatment	14
Diet Plan	14
A Diet for Diverticulitis Recovery	15
Percutaneous Drainage Using a CT Scan	18
Surgery	19
Chapter 2. What to Eat When Suffering From Diverticulitis	23
Food to Eat	23
Clear Liquid Diet for Diverticulitis	23
Low-Fiber Diet for Diverticulitis	24
Food to Avoid	24
Foods High in FODMAPs	24
Meats That Have Been Red and Processed	25
High-Sugar and High-Fat Foods	25
Shopping List	26
Chapter 3. Clear Liquid, Low Residue, and High Fiber	27
Phase 1: Clear Fluids (During a Flare)	27
Please Note	27
Phase 2: Low-Residue/Low-Fiber Diet (Immediately After a Controlled Flare)	28
Phase 3: High-Fiber Meals (Daily Life/Preventing Future Flares)	28
Breakfast	
Chapter 4. Clear Liquid Recipes	31
1. Fruit Punch	31
2. Chocolate Pudding	31
4. Oat Milk	32
3. Apple Juice	32
6. Black Tea	33
5. Cranberry Juice	33
8. Banana Almond Milk Smoothie	34
7. Mixed Berry Smoothie	34
9. Green Smoothie	35
10. Applesauce	35
Chapter 5. Low-Residue Recipes	37

    11. Greek Inspired Cucumber Salad — 37
    12. Light Veggie Salad — 37
    13. Eastern European Soup — 38
    14. Citrus Glazed Carrots — 38
    15. Spring Flavored Pasta — 39
    16. Gluten-Free Curry — 39
    17. Garden Veggies Quiche — 40
    18. Fluffy Pumpkin Pancakes — 40
    19. Sper-Tasty Chicken Muffins — 41
    20. Classic Zucchini Bread — 41

Chapter 6. High-Fiber Recipes — 43
    21. Pineapple Raspberry Parfaits — 43
    22. Berry Chia Pudding — 43
    23. Spinach Avocado Smoothie — 44
    24. Strawberry Pineapple Smoothie — 44
    25. Peach Blueberry Parfaits — 45
    26. Raspberry Yogurt Cereal Bowl — 45
    27. Avocado Toast — 46
    28. Loaded Pita Pockets — 46

Lunch recipes

Chapter 7. Clear Liquid Recipes — 49
    29. Grilled Vegetable Wrap Recipe with Hummus — 49
    30. Mediterranean Grilled Chicken Wrap — 49
    31. Green Goodness Sandwich — 50
    32. Turkey, Brie, and Apple Sandwich with Apple Cider Mayo — 50
    33. Black Beans and Cauliflower Rice (Gluten-Free, Vegan/Plant-Based) — 51
    34. Avocado Sauce Pasta — 52
    35. Greek Quinoa Bowls — 52
    36. Baked Sweet Potato Tacos — 53
    37. 5-Ingredient Sweet Potato Black Bean Chili — 53
    38. Whole-Wheat Pasta with Fresh Tomatoes and Herbs — 54
    39. Honey Mustard Salmon with Shaved Brussel Sprout Salad — 54
    40. 5-Minute Tomato Salad Lentil — 55

Chapter 8. Low-Residue Recipes — 57
    41. Veggies and Apple with Orange Sauce — 57
    42. Cauliflower Rice with Prawns and Veggies — 58
    43. Lentils with Tomatoes and Turmeric — 58
    44. Fried Rice with Kale — 59
    45. Stir-Fry Tofu and Red Pepper — 59
    46. Sweet Potato and Bell Pepper Hash with a Fried Egg — 60
    47. Quinoa Florentine — 60
    48. Tomato Asparagus Frittata — 61
    49. Shrimp and Mango Salsa Lettuce Wraps — 61
    50. Bacon-Wrapped Asparagus — 62
    51. Zucchini Pasta with Shrimp — 62
    52. Sweet Potato Buns Sandwich — 63
    53. Shrimp, Sausage, and Veggie Skillet — 64
    54. Sea Scallops with Spinach and Bacon — 64
    55. Liver with Onion and Parsley One — 65
    56. Egg and Avocado Wraps — 65
    57. Creamy Sweet Potato Pasta with Pancetta — 66
    58. Roasted Beet Pasta with Kale and Pesto — 67

Chapter 9. High-Fiber Recipes 69
59. Veggie Sandwich 69
60. Bean and Veggie Taco Bowl 69
61. Cobb Salad 70
62. Asparagus Soup 70
63. Lentil Soup 71
64. Mushroom Barley Soup 71
65. Broccoli Soup 72
66. Chicken and Asparagus Pasta 72
67. Red Beans and Rice 73
68. Beef Stir Fry 73
69. Black Bean Nacho Soup 74
70. Butternut Squash Soup 74
71. Broccoli Salad 75
72. Beef and Bean Sloppy Joes 75
73. Sweet Potato and Peanut Soup 76
74. Beet Salad 76
75. Broccoli Casserole 77

Dinner recipes

Chapter 10. Clear Liquid Recipes 81
76. Beet Soup 81
77. Chicken Burgers 81
78. Fresh Asparagus Soup 82
79. Pumpkin Waffles 82
80. Bean Soup 83
81. Carrot Cucumber Salad 83
82. Lemon Chicken and Rice 84
83. Peachy Pork with Rice 84
84. Loaded Pumpkin Chowder 85
85. Creamy Carrot Soup 85
86. Fish Stew 86
87. Mushroom Soup 86
88. Chicken Soup 87
89. Pumpkin Casserole 87
90. Fresh Tomato Juice 88
91. Ground Beef Tostada 88
92. Beef Barley Soup 89
93. Ground Beef and Rice Bowls 89

Chapter 11. Low-Residue Recipes 91
94. Grilled Vegetable Quesadilla 91
95. Grilled Veggie Sandwich 91
96. Lentil Linguine Stew 92
97. Lentil Risotto 92
98. Lentil Stew 93
99. Pasta with Beans and Turkey 93
100. Pasta with Spinach and White Beans 94
101. Chicken Florentine 94
102. Chipotle Black Bean Chili 95
103. Garnish with Fresh Cilantro 95
104. Couscous with Chicken 96
105. Couscous with Vegetables 96
106. Easy Beef Stir-Fry 97

107. Easy Turkey Chili	97
108. Garbanzo Pita Pockets	98
109. Grilled Fish Tacos	98
110. Grilled Steak with Spinach and Apple Salad	99

Chapter 12. High-Fiber Recipes — 101

111. Great Luncheon Salad	101
112. Flavors Powerhouse Lunch Meal	102
113. Eye-Catching Sweet Potato Boats	102
114. Mexican Enchiladas	103
115. Unique Banana Curry	103
116. Vegan-Friendly Platter	104
117. Armenian Style Chickpeas	104
118. Protein-Packed Soup	105
119. One-Pot Dinner Soup	105
120. 3-Beans Soup	106
121. Pork and Penne Pasta	106
122. Chicken and Quinoa Pita	107
123. Turkey Florentine	107
124. Chicken Lettuce Wraps	108
125. Couscous with Turkey	108
126. Ham, Bean, and Cabbage Stew	109

Snack and desserts recipes

Chapter 13. Clear Liquid Recipes — 113

127. Hummus with Tahini and Turmeric	113
128. Fiber Bars	113
129. Roasted Carrot Sticks in a Honey Garlic Marinade	114
130. Apple and Pistachio Salad on Spinach	114
131. Tomato Cashew Pesto	115
132. Sweet Potato Aioli	115
133. Eggplant Paste	116
134. Catalan Style Spinach	116

Chapter 14. Low-Residue Recipes — 119

135. Thai Coconut Lime Soup	119
136. Low-FODMAP French Oven Beef Stew	119
137. Veggie-Packed Low-FODMAP Soup	120
138. Cranberry Almond Oatmeal	121
139. Quick Banana Bread Oatmeal	121
140. Spicy Lemon Pasta with Shrimp	122
141. Chocolate Orange Chia Pudding	122
142. Fully Loaded Nachos	123

Chapter 15. High-Fiber Recipes — 125

143. Apricot Bars	125
144. Spaghetti Squash "Bolognese"	125
145. Lemon Sorbet	126
146. Raspberry and Lime Chia Parfait	126
147. Black Bean Hummus Crudité Platter	127
148. Celery Juice	128
149. Sweet Potato Chips	128
150. Guacamole	129

28-Day meal plan	131
Conclusion	135

Introduction

If you don't know what diverticulitis is, it's a condition that impacts more than 5 million Americans each year. It leads to inflammation of the rectum and colon, which can cause severe pain, cramping, diarrhea, and vomiting. A typical course of treatment may involve antibiotics or a diverticulitis diet.

Diverticular disease, including diverticulosis (a condition of having small pouches in the wall of the large intestine) and diverticulitis, is an inflammation of the colon (large intestine). Diversion disease refers to intestinal blockages. Diverticulitis, which occurs when a collection of inflammatory cells clogs up and obstructs the small intestine, is caused by a variety of factors such as faulty bacterial flora and a weakened immune system due to aging, smoking, or other causes.

Diverticulosis occurs when there are tiny dilated pouches in the muscular wall of your colon (small intestine) that are easily seen with a bowel movement.

Your intestinal tract is divided into the small intestine, which is where nutrients are absorbed, and the large intestine, which is where waste products are stored before they are excreted. Diverticulosis is a condition in which pouches, called diverticula, form in the wall of your colon. This small out-pouching can bulge through your intestinal wall that weakened as a result of recent surgeries or due to aging. The greatest percentage of these pouches occur amongst people over 60 years old. However, it may occur in younger people as well.

Diverticulitis occurs when one or more diverticula become inflamed or infected.

Your doctor may order imaging tests such as an upper GI series or a sigmoidoscopy to determine the state of your colon and your gastrointestinal tract in general. In addition, he or she might perform a colonoscopy to see if there are additional abnormalities that may need to be treated.

Treatment of diverticulitis involves taking medications to ease pain and swelling as well as antibiotics to treat the infection. If you have mild symptoms and no complications, your doctor may recommend rest and plenty of fluids. If your illness worsens or you develop complications, you should get medical help right once. In severe cases, surgery to clear blockages in your gut or repair a ruptured diverticulum may be required.

A diverticulitis diet includes supplements and other foods that can help strengthen the immune system, improve digestion and help treat the condition. For example, many nutritionists recommend taking vitamin C supplements to boost your immune system. It's also a good idea to increase your fiber intake because it aids in waste elimination. Your doctor can provide additional information on what foods to include in your diverticulitis diet and which ones to avoid. Following this diet closely is essential for managing your condition and preventing complications. If you're wondering how to proceed, talk to your doctor.

Chapter 1.
What Is Diverticulitis?

In older times, people used to have full grains, fibers, and lots of vegetables. Thus, digestive diseases were rare and often unheard of. Taking into account the huge change in the consumption patterns of people around the globe in the last century, such digestive diseases have become commonplace. People have adopted diets that are high in fat and sugar content. Such diets are devoid of essential nutrients and most importantly, the fibers that help in easy digestion and effective absorption of the nutrients.

Also, people do not take care of the liquid intake in the body and consume sodas and other drinks instead of plain replenishing water. A combination of a fiber-deficient diet along with a lack of water content in the body gives rise to conditions of constipation. People experience difficulty in passing on the stool, which gets stuck in the colon region giving rise to the condition of diverticulosis which later advances to a severe stage, called diverticulitis.

Vegetarians are the least affected by the disease since their diet is laden with fiber coming from grains, fruits, and vegetables. The non-vegetarians are at greater risk of contracting diverticulitis. Reports have it that the meat-eating western countries like America and the European nations have greater cases of the disease than the Asian countries where several of them have a vegetarian diet as their staple food. Africans have been the least affected by the disease because their diet is not as rich in fat.

Sedentary lifestyles and lack of exercise along with proper conditioning of the body add to the worsening of the condition. The disease is very difficult to diagnose in absence of any specific symptoms. It is often neglected in the earlier stages in lieu of ordinary digestive ailments and is not given much attention. The disease is progressive in nature and the situation deteriorates in absence of proper attentiveness.

Diverticulitis is a chronic digestive disease that involves the development of sacs or pouches in the bowel wall. These pouches are typically known as diverticula that appear on the sides of the longitudinal muscle surrounding the colon wall. This disease typically occurs in the colon or the large intestines. However, small intestines could also be affected by it.

Diverticulitis is the inflammation of one of these several diverticula. The inflammation can also be accompanied by an acute infection that is often detrimental to health. Diverticulitis in its milder forms is known as diverticulosis which is a commonly known medical condition. The most common symptoms a person with diverticulitis shows are excessive and continued pain in the lower abdominal region accompanied by fever and dizziness. The patient may also see a sizeable increase in the white blood cell count.

The most common reason for the development of the disease is assumed to be a fiber deficient diet. The disease is also associated with old age as the bowel system gets weaker as a person ages. Reports have it that almost all people above the age of 70 have been affected by diverticulitis.

Causes of Diverticulitis

Diverticulitis is caused by a variety of factors, with genetics accounting for about 40% of cases and environmental factors accounting for 60%. Another risk factor is obesity.

- **A diet low in fiber and heavy in animal fat.** Although the impact of low fiber alone is unclear, a low-fiber diet in combination with a high intake of animal fat appears to raise the risk.

- **Aging** Diverticulitis becomes more common as people get older.

- **Obesity.** You're more likely to get diverticulitis if you're severely overweight.

- **Smoking** People who smoke cigarettes are more prone to get diverticulitis than non-smokers.

- **A lack of physical activity.** Diverticulitis appears to be reduced by vigorous exercise.

- **A few drugs.** Several medicines, including steroids, opioids, and no steroidal anti-inflammatory drugs like ibuprofen (Advil, Motrin IB, and others), have been linked to an increased risk of diverticulitis (Aleve).

Symptoms of Diverticulitis

When the diverticula become inflamed, the symptoms of diverticulitis occur. These signs and symptoms include:

- Constant abdominal ache on the left side. It may appear on the right side in some circumstances.

- One of the most prevalent symptoms of diverticulitis is pain in the lower abdomen region. Nausea and fever are possible side effects. Diarrhea or constipation are other possible side effects.

- Diverticulosis can produce bleeding, which is usually painless.

- When you have bowel motions, bleeding from diverticulosis appears as bright red or maroon blood.

Please respond quickly if you observe any bleeding or pain in your abdomen.

If the infection is not treated quickly, diverticulitis can become an emergency. When the contents of your colon begin to seep into your abdominal cavity due to a perforation, it becomes an emergency (a tear). Diverticulitis bleeding usually goes away on its own, but it can be rather severe at times.

Your doctor may prescribe antibiotics for minor cases of diverticulitis. If you are bleeding, unable to take in fluids, or have severe aches or other symptoms, you may need to be admitted to the hospital.

If you have diverticulitis bleeding, you may need a colonoscopy while you're in the hospital. The doctor will be able to pinpoint the source of the bleeding using a colonoscopy. If there is no bleeding, you should undergo a colonoscopy as soon as the flare-up is over—that is if you haven't had one recently. The explanation for this is straightforward. Colon cancer often looks like diverticulitis, and it's an illness that needs to be treated as soon as possible.

Diarrhea, constipation, nausea, bloating, and cramping are some of the other symptoms of diverticular illness. Vomiting is a rare complication of diverticulitis. Your belly muscles reflexively contract up when your doctor applies pressure to your abdomen. Muscle defense is a reflex action that occurs as a result of this. If they suddenly let go, the pain will get worse.

Risk Factor

Diverticula form in weak sections of the intestine, according to research.

The origin is usually the sigmoid colon. The sigmoid colon is placed in front of the rectum and measures 40–45 cm in length. The strain on that muscle wall is caused by the contents of your intestine.

Genetics can also be a risk factor. Because of the nature of their DNA, certain people are more susceptible to developing this illness. Another risk factor includes weak connective tissue, as well as altered or troublesome wavelike movements of the intestinal wall. Diverticulitis is more likely to develop in those who are elderly or overweight.

Diverticulitis is influenced by lifestyle, but the extent of this influence has yet to be discovered. Constipation and the development of firm stools can be caused by a low-fiber diet. As a result, it stands to reason that a low-fiber meal can increase the risk of diverticular illness. Excessive red meat consumption, smoking, and not going to the bathroom regularly (having frequent movement) can all raise the risk.

The study of how the diverticulum becomes inflamed and the factors that increase the likelihood of this happening is still underway. Inflammation is more prone to occur in places with poor blood flow and in the diverticula where hard lumps of stool form.

People with a weaker immune system are more likely to develop complications, such as after severe renal disease or an organ transplant. Prolonged use of some medications, such as no steroidal anti-inflammatory drugs, acetylsalicylic acid, opiates, and steroids, increases the chance of more serious consequences.

Diverticulitis Associated Complications

An Abscess

Diverticulitis can cause infection, which usually clears itself after a few days of antibiotic treatment. An abscess in the colon wall may occur if the infection worsens.

An abscess is a collection of pus in a specific area that can cause swelling and tissue destruction. If the abscess is minor and remains in the colon's wall, antibiotic treatment may be enough to clear it out. If antibiotics do not clear up the abscess, the doctor may need to drain it with a catheter, which is a thin tube that is inserted into the abscess through the skin. The doctor inserts the needle through the skin until it reaches the abscess and then drains the fluid through the catheter after giving the patient numbing drugs. Sonography or x-ray may be used to guide this approach.

Perforation

Perforations can develop in infected diverticula. Peritonitis occurs when perforations in the colon allow us to flow out and develop a big abscess in the abdominal cavity. Peritonitis can make a person very sick, causing nausea, vomiting, fever, and acute abdominal tenderness. The illness necessitates prompt surgery to clear the abdominal cavity and eliminate the colon damage. Peritonitis can be lethal if not treated quickly.

Bleeding in the Rectal Area

Diverticula-related rectal bleeding is a rare complication. Doctors believe the bleeding is caused by a weakening and eventually bursting of a tiny blood vessel in a diverticulum. When the diverticula bleed, blood may appear in the toilet or the stool. Although bleeding might be significant, it often stops on its own and does not require treatment. If you have rectum bleeding, even if it's only a small quantity, you should consult a doctor right away. Colonoscopy is frequently performed to pinpoint the source of bleeding and stop it. To diagnose and treat diverticular bleeding, the doctor may inject dye into an artery, a procedure known as angiography. If the bleeding does not cease, surgery to remove the affected part of the colon may be required.

Fistula

A fistula is a tissue connection between 2 organs or between an organ and the abnormal skin. When infected tissues come into contact with one another, they can sometimes cling together. A fistula may occur if they heal this way. The colon's tissue may attach to surrounding tissues if a diverticulitis-related illness extends outside the colon. The bladder, small intestine, and skin are the most commonly affected organs.

Fistulas between the bladder and the colon are the most prevalent. Men are more likely than women to develop this sort of fistula. It can lead to a serious and long-lasting urinary tract infection. Surgery to remove the fistula and the damaged section of the colon can solve the condition.

Obstruction of the Intestines

Intestinal obstruction occurs when scarring produced by infection causes a partial or complete blockage of the gut. The colon is unable to move stool contents normally when the gut is clogged. Emergency surgery is required if the intestine is fully obstructed. Because partial blockage is not an emergency, surgery to correct it can be scheduled ahead of time.

Options for Diverticulitis Treatment

Diet Plan

A low residue diet may be prescribed. A low-fiber diet was formerly assumed to allow the colon enough time to heal. The evidence contradicts this, with a 2011 analysis showing no evidence for the efficacy of low residue diets in the treatment of diverticular disease and suggesting that a high-fiber diet may help avoid the condition. Although no high-quality research was discovered in a systematic review published in 2012, various studies and guidelines favored a high-fiber diet for the treatment of symptomatic illness.

A Diet for Diverticulitis Recovery

It's critical to help your digestive tract clean itself out and mend during a diverticulitis flare-up, or at the onset of symptoms. Use my beef bone broth recipe as a starting point.

Eating bone broths prepared from cattle, chicken, lamb, and fish aids in the healing of leaky gut syndrome, improve joint health, strengthens the immune system, and even helps to reduce cellulite, all while aiding in the healing of the digestive tract.

Bone broths, when combined with cooked vegetables and a small amount of meat, offer your body critical minerals such as calcium, magnesium, phosphorus, silicon, sulfur, and more, in an easily digestible form.

Vegetables such as carrots, celery, and garlic, as well as an egg poached in the soup, can be added to your bone broth. In addition, drink 2–3 cups of warm ginger tea each day to help reduce inflammation and assist digestion. Ginger is a nutrient-dense spice that boosts your immune and digestive systems.

The collagen in the bones of cattle and chicken breaks down into gelatin in roughly 48 hours and 24 hours, respectively. Although you may prepare broth in less time, I recommend cooking it in a crockpot for at least 48 hours to extract the most flavor out of the bones.

Gelatin has incredible healing powers, and it can even help people with food sensitivities and allergies handle these foods better. It also helps to maintain a healthy probiotic balance by breaking down proteins to make them easier to digest. The truth about probiotics is that they aid in the creation of a healthy gut environment.

Only clear bone broths, clear fresh juices (no pulp), and soothing ginger tea should be consumed during the first phase of the diverticulitis diet.

Start adding fiber-rich foods like fresh fruits and vegetables, as well as unprocessed grains like quinoa, black rice, fermented grains, or sprouted lentils, once your body has adjusted to these foods.

Whole nuts and seeds should be avoided since they can easily become trapped in the diverticula and cause more harm.

Fiber, according to University of Oxford experts, lowers the incidence of diverticular illness. Fiber from fruits, vegetables, grains, and potatoes was studied.

So, gradually introduce high-fiber foods throughout the first several days, introducing one new food every 3–4 days.

As your body adjusts, start taking about 25–35 g of fiber per day to help prevent any potential flare-ups while your digestive tract repairs. Start with potatoes, sweet potatoes, and root vegetables, and then gradually include non-processed grains and beans like oats and lentils.

The distinction between soluble and insoluble fiber is one of the most significant distinctions to make. Soluble fiber absorbs water and transforms into a gel as it passes through the digestive system. The gel aids digestion by slowing it down, enabling more critical nutrients to be absorbed. Insoluble fiber, on the other hand, bulks up stools, allowing food to pass through your system more rapidly.

Oat bran, nuts, seeds, beans, lentils, barley, and peas are all high in soluble fiber.

Whole grains, wheat bran, and vegetables are all high in insoluble fiber.

Researchers from Harvard Medical School's Department of Nutrition discovered that insoluble fiber lowers the likelihood of developing diverticular disease. But don't let this deter you from maintaining a healthy diet. You don't have to, and you shouldn't, avoid soluble fiber.

Diverticulitis can flare up if a proper balance of protein, fiber, and fresh fruits and vegetables is not maintained.

For millennia, Native Americans have used slippery elm both topically and internally to ease stomach disorders, coughs, and sore throats.

It is now advised for the relief of GERD, Crohn's disease, IBS, and digestive upset symptoms.

Begin by taking 500 milligrams 3 times a day for the duration of the diverticulitis diet. Make sure you drink a full glass of water or another clear liquid before taking this supplement.

Aloe juice assists digestion, normalizes pH levels, regulates the intestinal function and promotes the growth of good digestive bacteria. Aloe vera juice containing "aloe latex" should be avoided because it might induce severe stomach cramps and diarrhea.

Aloe juice in the amount of ½–16 oz per day is advised; any more than that will irritate your system.

It's in the organics area of your local grocery store, as well as many Asian stores.

Licorice root reduces stomach acid, relieves heartburn, and acts as a mild laxative to aid in the elimination of waste from the colon. This root aids digestion by increasing bile production and decreasing cholesterol levels. When you have symptoms of diverticulitis, take 100 milligrams every day.

The ultimate purpose of the diverticulitis diet, vitamins, and lifestyle adjustments is to encourage your digestive tract to work efficiently, in addition to repairing your colon from diverticulitis.

Digestive enzymes aid in the breakdown of foods, allowing nutrients to be absorbed. Individuals with digestive issues might take digestive supplements containing vital enzymes to help with digestion.

Live probiotics should be included in one's diet to help with food sensitivities and digestive issues such as constipation, gas, and bloating Probiotics are beneficial bacteria that line the lining of the digestive tract and aid in infection resistance. If you have diverticulitis, you need an infusion of these bacteria to help repair your colon and avoid the recurrence of the disease.

Diverticulitis necessitates more than just a diverticulitis diet and supplements to keep the digestive tract healthy. The mouth is where digestion begins. It is critical to chew each bite of food thoroughly until it is virtually liquefied. The more food is broken down before it reaches the stomach, the more nutrients are available for absorption.

Diverticular illness can be prevented by combining physical exercise and a high-fiber diet, according to medical studies. Running or utilizing a rebounder daily can help ease symptoms and flare-ups. Even moderate-intensity exercise aids in bowel function regulation, stress reduction, and weight management.

Your psychological well-being is intertwined with your physical well-being; stress management and the development of efficient coping mechanisms are critical. Stress has an impact on both the mind and the body.

When you strain on the toilet, you put too much pressure on your colon, which causes minor tears.

Choose a stool that allows you to elevate your feet slightly to decrease strain.

Antibiotics

Diverticulitis can cause infection, which usually clears itself after a few days of antibiotic treatment. An abscess in the colon wall may occur if the infection worsens.

An abscess is a collection of pus in a specific area that can cause swelling and tissue destruction. If the abscess is minor and remains in the colon's wall, antibiotic treatment may be enough to clear it out. If antibiotics do not clear up the abscess, the doctor may need to drain it with a catheter, which is a thin tube that is inserted into the abscess through the skin. The doctor inserts the needle through the skin until it reaches the abscess and then drains the fluid through the catheter after giving the patient numbing drugs. Sonography or x-ray may be used to guide this approach.

Percutaneous Drainage Using a CT Scan

CT scans are routinely used to examine people who have the symptoms listed above.

The use of a CT scan to diagnose diverticulitis is extremely accurate (98 percent). Thin section (5 mm) transverse pictures are taken through the entire belly and pelvis after the patient has been given oral and intravascular contrast to extract as much information as possible regarding the patient's health. The images show localized thickening of the colon wall, as well as inflammation that has spread to the fat around the colon. When the affected segment contains diverticula, an accurate diagnosis of acute diverticulitis can be obtained. Patients with more serious diverticulitis, such as those who have an accompanying abscess, may be identified using CT scans. It might even allow for radiologically guided abscess draining, avoiding the need for emergency surgery.

The doctor will ask about your medical history, perform a physical exam, and maybe order one or more diagnostic tests to determine whether you have diverticular disease. Diverticulosis is frequently discovered through testing requested for a different condition because most patients have no symptoms. Diverticulosis, for example, is frequently discovered during a colonoscopy, which is performed to check for cancer or polyps, as well as to assess complaints of pain or rectal bleeding

Doctors may inquire about bowel habits, discomfort, other symptoms, nutrition, and medications when collecting a medical history. A digital rectal exam is typically part of the physical examination. The doctor uses a gloved, lubricated finger to detect pain, obstruction, or blood in the rectum. The doctor may check for evidence of bleeding in the stool and perform a blood test to look for signs of infection.

A CT scan is a type of imaging that uses a computer to create a 3-dimensional image of the body. A CT scan is a non-invasive x-ray that generates cross-section images of the body. The doctor may inject dye into a vein and administer a comparable combination for the patient to drink. The person is lying on a table that slips inside a machine that looks like a donut.

The dye aids in the detection of problems like perforations and abscesses that might occur as a result of diverticulitis.

Surgery

A hospital stay will almost certainly be required in severe cases of diverticulitis with intense pain and consequences. Surgery may be required if a patient develops problems or fails to respond to therapy.

Perforations can form in infected diverticula. Peritonitis is a disorder that occurs when perforations in the colon allow us to flow out and build a big abscess in the abdominal cavity. Nausea, vomiting, fever, and acute abdominal discomfort are common symptoms of peritonitis. The situation necessitates prompt surgery to clear the abdominal cavity and remove the colon section that has been injured. Peritonitis can be lethal if not treated promptly.

Diverticula-related rectal bleeding is a rather uncommon side effect. The bleeding is thought to be triggered by a weakening and then bursting of a tiny blood artery in a diverticulum. Blood can occur in the toilet or in the stool when the diverticula bleed. Bleeding can be significant, but it often stops on its own and does not require medical attention. Any rectum bleeding, no matter how minor, should be seen by a doctor as soon as possible. Colonoscopy is frequently performed to locate and control bleeding in the colon. To identify and treat diverticular bleeding, the doctor may inject dye into an artery, a procedure known as angiography. If the bleeding persists, surgery to remove the affected part of the colon may be required.

A fistula between the bladder and the colon is the most common type of fistula. Men are more likely than women to have this sort of fistula. It can cause a serious, long-term urinary tract infection. Surgery to remove the fistula and the damaged portion of the colon can be used to repair the condition.

Infection-related scarring can result in intestinal obstruction, which is a partial or complete blockage of the intestine. The colon is unable to transport bowel contents normally when the gut becomes clogged. Emergency surgery may be required if the intestine is fully obstructed. The operation to correct a partial blockage is not an emergency, thus it can be scheduled.

- Surgery's Risks

There are risks and potential consequences associated with every procedure. You should talk to your doctor about all of the possible hazards.

- After the Surgery: What to Expect

There are risks and potential consequences associated with every procedure. All dangers and healing should be discussed with your physician.

- Expectations and Requirements After Discharge

There are risks and potential consequences associated with every procedure. All dangers and healing should be discussed with your doctor.

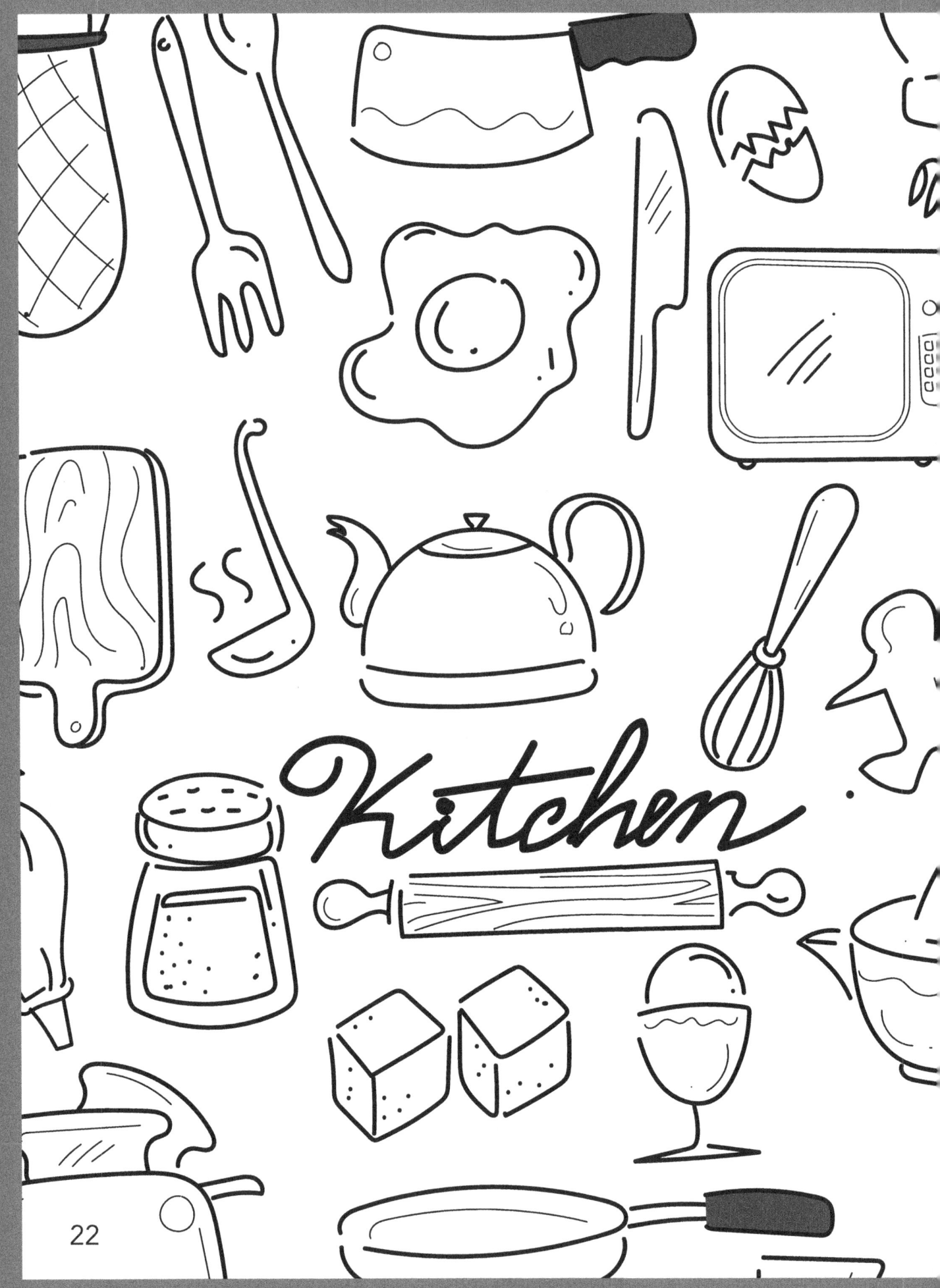

Chapter 2.
What to Eat When Suffering From Diverticulitis

Food to Eat

"On the other hand, when you have diverticulitis, your polyps become irritated, inflamed, and possibly infected." Taylor explains, "We aim to lessen traffic in your GI tract so that nothing else disturbs them. Reducing the amount of fiber in your diet can assist."

During a flare-up of diverticulitis, your doctor may advise rest, antibiotics, and a clear liquid or low-fiber diet.

Clear Liquid Diet for Diverticulitis

A clear liquid diet may be recommended if a diverticulitis flare-up is severe or necessitates surgery. "You graduate from clear liquids to a low-fiber diet after 1–2 days," Taylor explains. "Even if your pain does not go away, you continue to eat usual foods. You can't stay on a liquid diet for an extended period of time because you'll get malnourished."

You can eat the following foods on a clear liquid diet:

- Broths that are clear (not soup).

- Juices that are clear and pulp-free (such as apple and cranberry juice)

- Popsicles

- Water

Low-Fiber Diet for Diverticulitis

Eat a low-fiber, or GI soft, diet for milder forms of diverticulitis. Depending on the severity of the flare-up, a low-fiber diet restricts fiber consumption to 8 ½ g per day.

Low-fiber foods to consider include:

- **Grains:** White spaghetti and white bread lovers, rejoice! These, as well as white rice and white crackers, are low-fiber options.

- **Starches with low-fiber content:** Take out your peeler. Potatoes with no skin are an option. They can be mashed, roasted, or baked. Corn flakes and puffed rice cereal are 2 low-fiber kinds of cereal that get a thumbs up.

- **Eggs and egg whites, tofu, and meat or seafood are all good sources of protein.** "Shredded chicken, lean ground beef, and soft baked fish are the finest choices."

- **Fruits:** Be cautious when eating fruits because they contain a lot of fiber. Canned fruits like peaches and pears, applesauce, ripe bananas, and soft, ripe cantaloupe and honeydew are all good choices. "You're not eating the skin, so there's not a lot of fiber." Insoluble fiber, which can irritate inflamed polyps, is found in the skins."

- **If you're recovering from a flare-up, cottage cheese, and Greek yogurt are big winners:** They're high in protein, calcium, and other nutrients, plus they don't have any fiber. They're also soft, moist, and easier to swallow if you're sick. Milk and cheeses are also options.

Food to Avoid

Foods High in FODMAPs

Some persons with irritable bowel syndrome benefit from following a low FODMAP diet (IBS). Some persons with diverticulitis may benefit from it as well.

FODMAPs are carbohydrate types. Fermentable oligosaccharides, disaccharides, monosaccharides, and polyols are all included.

People who follow this diet avoid foods that are rich in FODMAPS. This includes, for example, the following foods:

- Apples, pears, and plums are examples of fruits.

- Fermented foods, such as sauerkraut or kimchi beans dairy foods, such as milk, yogurt, and ice cream.

- Legumes.

- Meals with a lot of trans fats.

- Cabbage with soy sauce.

- Brussels sprouts.

- Garlic and onions.

Meats That Have Been Red and Processed

Eating a diet strong in red and processed meats may raise your chance of having diverticulitis. A diet rich in fruits, vegetables, and whole grains may help to lower the risk of heart disease.

High-Sugar and High-Fat Foods

The typical Western diet is high in fat, sugar, and fiber, but low in fiber. As a result, a person's risk of having diverticulitis may increase.

According to a 2017 study with over 46,000 male participants, avoiding the following foods may help prevent or lessen the symptoms of diverticulitis:

Fried food, red meat, refined carbohydrates, full-fat dairy.

Shopping List

Your doctor will most likely recommend that you gradually start shopping for solid foods after your symptoms have subsided. Begin by consuming low-fiber, readily digestible foods like dairy, eggs, low-fiber cereal and bread, pasta, white rice, and canned or soft fruits and vegetables with no seeds or skin. Gradually increase your fiber intake by 5–15 g per day until you can eat a high-fiber diet once more.

Chapter 3.
Clear Liquid, Low Residue, and High Fiber

There are three main phases of the diverticulitis diet: eating during an active flare-up, eating while recovering from a flare, and preventing a flare in the future. As with any other diet, you will need to listen to your body throughout each stage and adjust the diet slowly as you add new foods while closely monitoring your symptoms.

Phase 1: Clear Fluids (During a Flare)

While going through an active flare, your symptoms can become extreme. Due to this, it's smart for you to give your bowel a period of rest. As you can imagine the best way to do this is by sticking to a clear fluid diet. This will aid in your recovery as your body may outright reject solid foods.

It is vital to note that the clear fluid stage of the diet is not intended to be a long-term diet. In fact, the general expectation is that you remain in this stage for no more than a couple of days.

Please Note

Restricting yourself to a clear fluid diet for an excessive amount of time may cause you to feel light-headed, weak, hungry, and fatigued. You can also experience muscle wasting, excessive weight loss, and depletion of vitamins and minerals.

This occurs because it's incredibly difficult to meet the body's daily caloric requirements for fat, protein, and carbohydrates through a clear fluid diet. The average person will need to provide their body with at least 200 grams of carbohydrates to have enough energy to go through the day. If you struggle with low blood sugar, diabetes, or other blood sugar challenges, you may want to monitor your blood sugar levels during this stage.

As the name implies, this phase is composed of clear liquids. These include green tea, fresh fruit juice, clear broth, and gelatin dessert. The clear liquid diet provides the body with salt, liquids, and enough nutrients to function temporarily, generally for a few days, until you can eat normal food.

Phase 2: Low-Residue/Low-Fiber Diet (Immediately After a Controlled Flare)

A low-residue (or low-fiber) diet acts as the reintroduction phase, after your flare-up symptoms have mostly passed but before your body is ready for high-fiber or high residue foods.

Phase 3: High-Fiber Meals (Daily Life/Preventing Future Flares)

This final stage in the diverticulitis diet is the high fiber diet. This stage is used to maintain a balanced diet while preventing a future flare. It is basically your general day-to-day eating routineand generally takes up the majority of your diverticulitis eating plan.

It is important to note, however, that you do not want to jump directly from a significantly low fiber diet (such as a clear fluid diet) directly to a high fiber diet, as this will do more harm to your colon than good. It is always best to ease into any stage of the plan that requires an increase in your fiber intake. Aim to increase your fiber intake by 2–4 g per week until you reach the recommended amount for your age and biology. Bear in mind that as you increase your fiber, you also need to increase your water intake to help move the fiber through your intestinal tract.

Breakfast

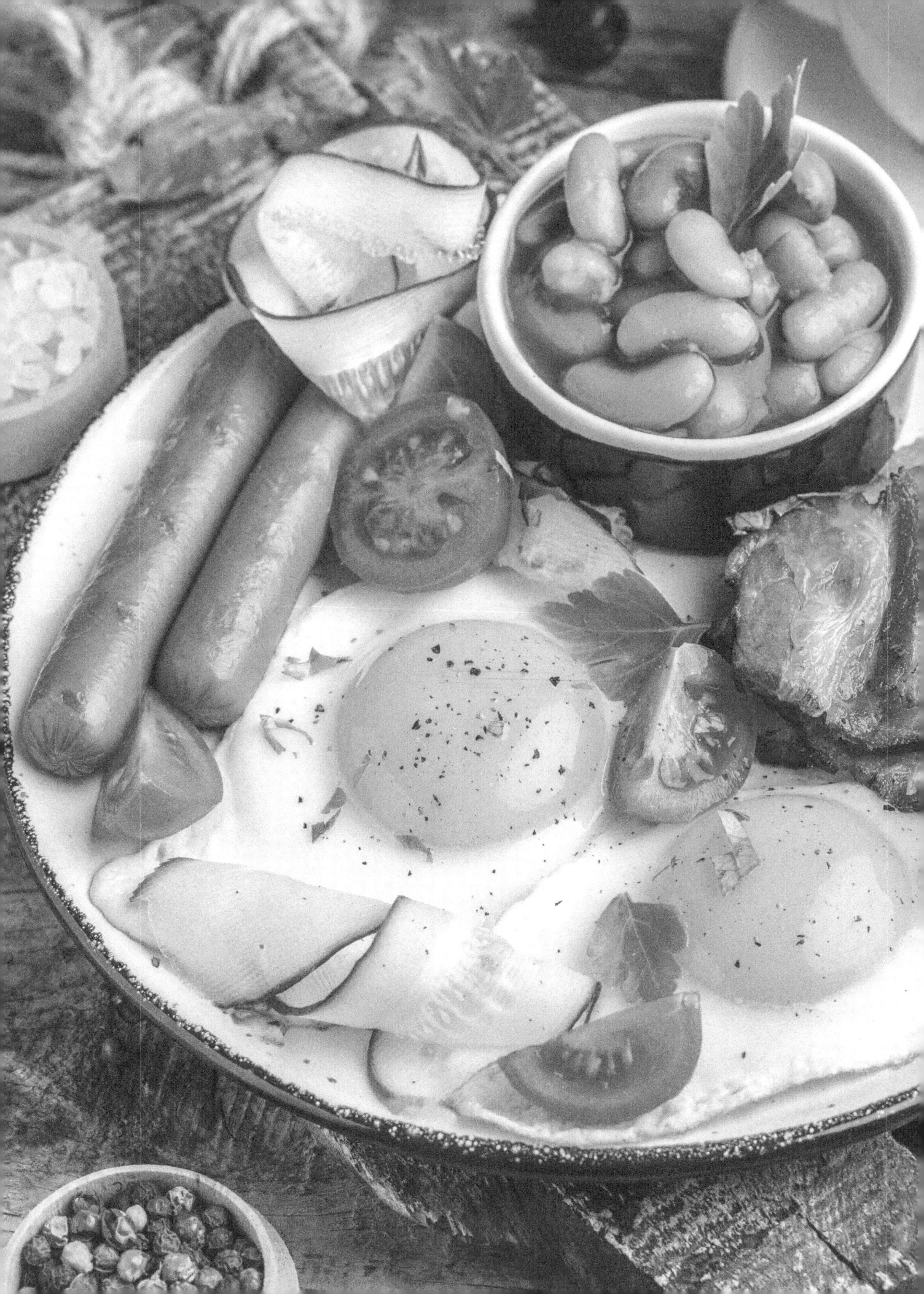

Chapter 4. Clear Liquid Recipes

Preparation time: 10 minutes
Cooking time: 0 minutes
Servings: 10

1. Fruit Punch

INGREDIENTS
- 4 cups cranberry juice
- 1 ½ cup pineapple juice
- 1 ½ cup orange juice
- ¼ cup lime juice
- 3 cups chilled ginger ale

DIRECTIONS
1. Add lime juice, orange juice, cranberry juice, and pineapple juice into the pitcher and chill for 1 hour.
2. Add ginger ale and stir well.

NUTRITION
- Calories: 39
- Carbs: 9 g
- Fat: 0.1 g
- Proteins: 1 g

Preparation time: 10 minutes
Cooking time: 0 minutes
Servings: 8

2. Chocolate Pudding

INGREDIENTS
- 1 cup sugar
- ½ cup baking cocoa
- ¼ cup cornstarch
- ½ tsp salt
- 4 cups dairy-free milk, such as oat milk and almond milk
- 2 tbsp dairy-free butter
- 2 tsp vanilla extract

DIRECTIONS
1. Mix the salt, cornstarch, cocoa, and sugar into the saucepan. Add dairy-free milk gradually. Bring to a boil over medium flame, about 2 minutes.
2. Remove from the flame. Add dairy-free butter and vanilla extract and stir well.
3. Pour pudding into the bowl. Let it chill until ready to serve!

NUTRITION
- Calories: 196
- Carbohydrates 38 g
- Fat: 4 g
- Proteins: 5 g

Preparation time: 1 minute
Cooking time: 0 minutes
Servings: 4

3. Apple Juice

INGREDIENTS
- 8 apples, washed and peeled
- 3 tbsp sugar

DIRECTIONS
1. Rinse and peel the apples. Cut into chunks. Remove seeds.
2. Add apple chunks and sugar into the juicer and blend until smooth.
3. Serve and enjoy!

NUTRITION
- Calories: 114
- Fat: 0.3 g
- Carbohydrate: 28 g
- Protein: 0.3 g

Preparation time: 10 minutes
Cooking time: 0 minutes
Servings: 8

4. Oat Milk

INGREDIENTS
- 1 cup rolled oats
- 4 cups cold water
- 1-2 tbsp optional maple syrup
- 1 tsp vanilla extract
- A pinch of salt

DIRECTIONS
1. Firstly, add oats, water, and maple syrup into the blender. Blend for 20–30 seconds.
2. Strain oat milk mixture with cheesecloth or strainer over a big mixing bowl. Discard solid parts.
3. Serve and enjoy!

NUTRITION
- Calories: 19
- Carbs: 3 g
- Fat: 1 g
- Proteins: 1 g

5. Cranberry Juice

Preparation time: 10 minutes
Cooking time: 0 minutes
Servings: 8

INGREDIENTS

- 2 cups cranberries
- 2 cups pure water
- 1 ½ tbsp lemon juice
- 1 tsp honey

DIRECTIONS

1. Add cranberries and water into the blender and blend at high speed for 2 minutes.
2. Pass the juice through a strainer or cheesecloth and remove solid pieces.
3. Add lemon juice and honey to the juice.
4. When done, serve it into the glasses.

NUTRITION

- Calories: 3
- Carbs: 1 g
- Fat: 1 g
- Proteins: 1 g

---

6. Black Tea

Preparation time: 5 minutes
Cooking time: 5 minutes
Servings: 2

INGREDIENTS

- 2 cups water
- ½ tsp tea
- Sugar to taste

DIRECTIONS

1. Add water into the pot and boil it.
2. Then, add tea and turn off the flame.
3. Cover the pot with a lid and keep it aside for 2–3 minutes.
4. Add sugar into the serving cups, and then add tea.
5. Serve and enjoy!

NUTRITION

- Calories: 2.4
- Carbs: 0.4 g
- Fat: 0 g
- Proteins: 0.1 g

Preparation time: 5 minutes
Cooking time: 0 minutes
Servings: 2

7. Mixed Berry Smoothie

INGREDIENTS

- ½ cup dairy-free yogurt
- 12 oz frozen mixed berries
- 1 tbsp honey

DIRECTIONS

- Add dairy-free yogurt, honey, and mixed berries into the blender and blend until smooth.
- Pour smoothie into the glass.
- Serve and enjoy!

NUTRITION

- Calories: 171
- Carbs: 38 g
- Fat: 2 g
- Proteins: 4 g

Preparation time: 5 minutes
Cooking time: 0 minutes
Servings: 2

8. Banana Almond Milk Smoothie

INGREDIENTS

- 2 bananas, sliced and frozen
- 1 cup almond milk
- 1 tbsp flax seeds
- 1 tsp vanilla extract
- ½ tsp cinnamon

DIRECTIONS

1. Mix all ingredients into the blender and blend until smooth.
2. Serve and enjoy!

NUTRITION

- Calories: 312
- Carbs: 59 g
- Fat: 8 g
- Proteins: 5 g

Preparation time: 5 minutes
Cooking time: 0 minutes
Servings: 1

9. Green Smoothie

INGREDIENTS

- 1 cup water or milk, such as almond or hemp milk
- ½ cup orange juice
- 1-2 big handfuls of fresh baby spinach
- 1 frozen banana, cut into coins
- 1 mango, frozen
- 1 tbsp almond butter or peanut butter
- ¼ avocado, peeled and pit removed

DIRECTIONS

1. Add water, spinach, and orange juice into the blender and blend until broken down.
2. Add peanut butter or almond butter and blend until smooth.
3. Then, add frozen mango and banana and blend until smooth.
4. Serve and enjoy!

NUTRITION

- Calories: 267
- Carbs: 66 g
- Fat: 1 g
- Proteins: 4 g

Preparation time: 5 minutes
Cooking time: 20 minutes
Servings: 4

10. Applesauce

INGREDIENTS

- 4 Bramley apples, peeled and diced into small chunks
- 4 tbsp brown sugar
- ½ juice only lemon
- ½ tbsp dairy-free butter
- A pinch of ground cinnamon

DIRECTIONS

1. Add sugar, lemon juice, and apple into the pot. Place it over medium-low flame.
2. Add cinnamon, dairy-free butter, and sugar and stir well.

NUTRITION

- Calories: 70
- Carbs: 16.9 g
- Fat: 0.79 g
- Protein: 0.35 g

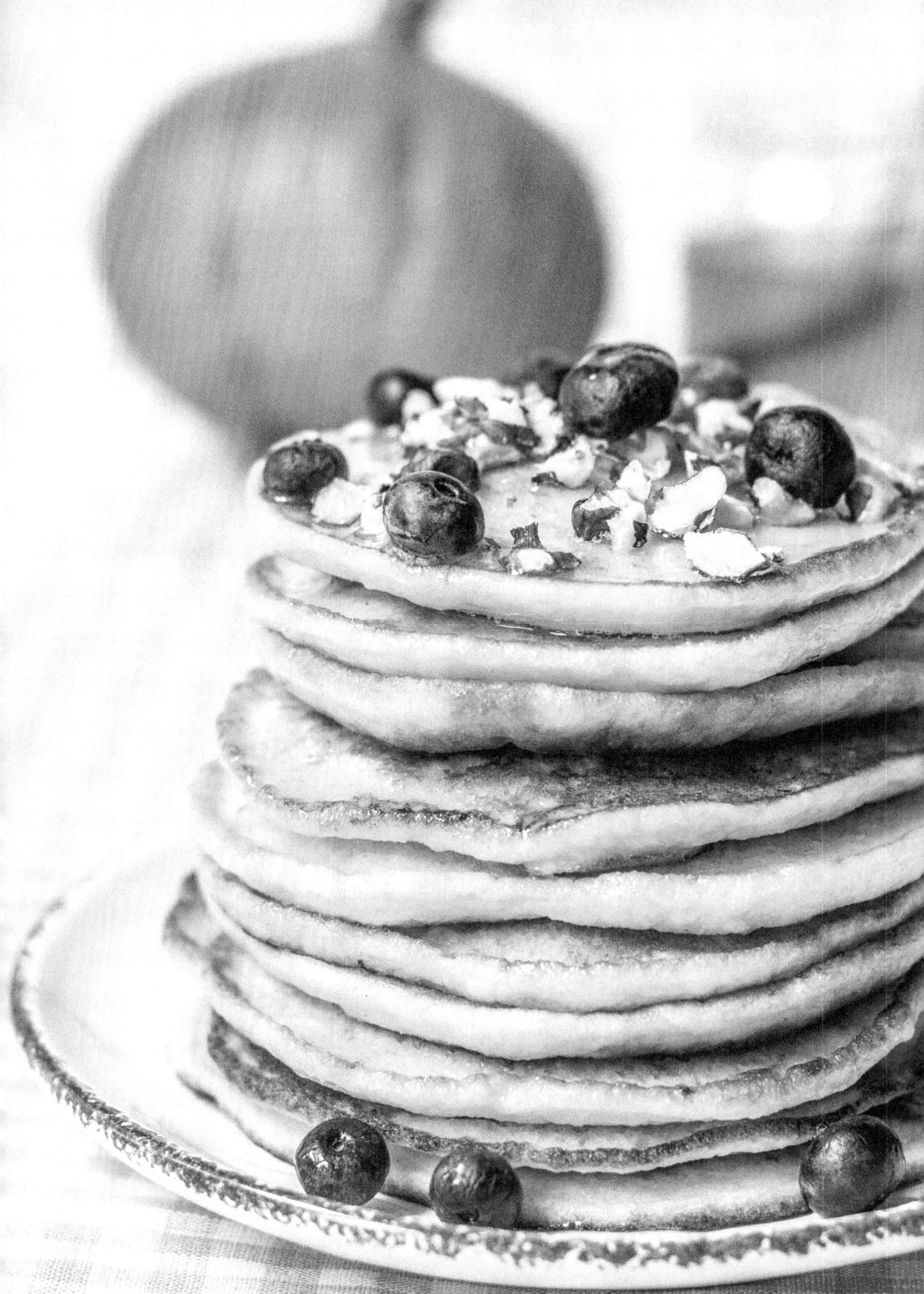

Chapter 5. Low-Residue Recipes

11. Greek Inspired Cucumber Salad

Preparation time: 10 minutes
Cooking time: 0 minutes
Servings: 4

INGREDIENTS

- 4 medium cucumbers, peeled, seeded, and chopped
- ½ cup low-fat Greek yogurt
- 1 ½ tbsp fresh dill, chopped
- 1 tbsp fresh lemon juice
- Salt and freshly ground black pepper, as required

DIRECTIONS

1. In a large bowl, add all the ingredients and mix well.
2. Serve immediately.

NUTRITION

- Calories: 71
- Carbs: 13.8 g
- Protein: 4 g
- Fat: 0.8 g
- Sugar: 7.3 g
- Sodium: 69 mg
- Fiber: 1.7 g

---

12. Light Veggie Salad

Preparation time: 10 minutes
Cooking time: 0 minutes
Servings: 5

INGREDIENTS

- 2 cups cucumbers, peeled, seeded, and chopped
- 2 cups red tomatoes, peeled, seeded, and chopped
- 2 tbsp extra-virgin olive oil
- 2 tbsp fresh lime juice
- Salt to taste

DIRECTIONS

1. In a large serving bowl, add all the ingredients and toss to coat well.
2. Serve immediately.

NUTRITION

- Calories: 68
- Carbs: 04.4 g
- Protein: 0.9 g
- Fat: 5.8 g
- Sugar: 2.6 g
- Sodium: 35 mg
- Fiber: 1.1 g

Preparation time: 10 minutes
Cooking time: 5 minutes
Servings: 3

13. Eastern European Soup

INGREDIENTS

- 2 cups fat-free yogurt
- 4 tsp fresh lemon juice
- 2 cups beets, trimmed, peeled, and chopped
- 2 tbsp fresh dill
- Salt as required
- 1 tbsp fresh chives, minced

DIRECTIONS

1. In a high-speed blender, add all ingredients except for chives and pulse until smooth.
2. Transfer the soup into a pan over medium heat and cook for about 3–5 minutes or until heated through.
3. Serve immediately with the garnishing of chives.

NUTRITION

- Calories: 149
- Carbs: 25.2 g
- Protein: 11.8 g
- Fat: 0.6 g
- Sugar: 21.7 g
- Sodium: 269 mg
- Fiber: 2.5 g

Preparation time: 15 minutes
Cooking time: 15 minutes
Servings: 6

14. Citrus Glazed Carrots

INGREDIENTS

- 1 ½ lb carrots, peeled and sliced into ½-inch pieces diagonally
- ½ cup water
- 2 tbsp olive oil
- Salt to taste
- 3 tbsp fresh orange juice

DIRECTIONS

1. In a large skillet, add the carrots, water, boil, and salt over medium heat and bring to a boil.
2. Reduce heat to low and simmer; covered for about 6 minutes.
3. Add the orange juice and stir to combine.
4. Increase the heat to high and cook, uncovered for about 5–8 minutes, tossing frequently.
5. Serve immediately.

NUTRITION

- Calories: 90
- Carbs: 12 g
- Protein: 1 g
- Fat: 4.7 g
- Sugar: 6.2 g
- Sodium: 106 mg
- Fiber: 2.8 g

15. Spring Flavored Pasta

Preparation time: 10 minutes
Cooking time: 10 minutes
Servings: 4

INGREDIENTS

- 2 tbsp olive oil
- 1 lb asparagus, trimmed and cut into 1½-inch piece
- Salt and freshly ground black pepper, to taste
- ½ lb cooked hot pasta, drained

DIRECTIONS

1. In a large cast-iron skillet, heat the oil over medium heat and cook the asparagus, salt, and black pepper for about 8-10 minutes, stirring occasionally.
2. Place the hot pasta and toss to coat well.
3. Serve immediately.

NUTRITION

- Calories: 246
- Carbs: 35.2 g
- Protein: 8.9 g
- Fat: 8.4 g
- Sugar: 2.1 g
- Sodium: 17 mg
- Fiber: 2.4 g

---

16. Gluten-Free Curry

Preparation time: 15 minutes
Cooking time: 20 minutes
Servings: 6

INGREDIENTS

- 2 cups tomatoes, peeled, seeded, and chopped
- 1 ½ cup water
- 2 tbsp olive oil
- 1 tsp fresh ginger, chopped
- ¼ tsp ground turmeric
- 2 cups fresh shiitake mushrooms, sliced
- 5 cups fresh button mushrooms, sliced
- ¼ cup fat-free yogurt, whipped
- Salt and freshly ground black pepper to taste

DIRECTIONS

1. In a food processor, add the tomatoes and ¼ cup of water and pulse until a smooth paste forms.
2. In a pan, heat the oil over medium heat and sauté the ginger and turmeric for about 1 minute.
3. Add the tomato paste and cook for about 5 minutes.
4. Stir in the mushrooms, yogurt, and remaining water and bring to a boil.
5. Cook for about 10-12 minutes, stirring occasionally.
6. Season with salt and black pepper and remove from the heat.
7. Serve hot.

NUTRITION

- Calories: 70
- Carbs: 5.3 g
- Protein: 3 g
- Fat: 5 g
- Sugar: 3.4 g
- Sodium: 41 mg
- Fiber: 1.4 g

17. Garden Veggies Quiche

Preparation time: 15 minutes
Cooking time: 20 minutes
Servings: 4

INGREDIENTS

- 6 eggs
- ½ cup low-fat milk
- Salt and freshly ground black pepper, to taste
- 2 cups fresh baby spinach, chopped
- ½ cup green bell pepper, seeded and chopped
- 1 scallion, chopped
- ¼ cup fresh parsley, chopped
- 1 tbsp fresh chives, minced

DIRECTIONS

1. Preheat the oven to 400°F. Lightly grease a pie dish.
2. In a bowl, add eggs, almond milk, salt, and black pepper and beat until well combined. Set aside.
3. In another bowl, add the vegetables and herbs and mix well.
4. In the bottom of a prepared pie dish, place the veggie mixture evenly and top with the egg mixture.
5. Bake for about 20 minutes or until a wooden skewer inserted in the center comes out clean.
6. Remove the pie dish from the oven and set it aside for about 5 minutes before slicing
7. Cut into desired-sized wedges and serve warm.

NUTRITION

- Calories: 118
- Carbs: 4.3 g
- Protein: 10.1 g
- Fat: 7 g
- Sugar: 3 g
- Sodium: 160 mg
- Fiber: 0.8 g

---

18. Fluffy Pumpkin Pancakes

Preparation time: 10 minutes
Cooking time: 40 minutes
Servings: 10

INGREDIENTS

- 2 eggs
- 1 cup buckwheat flour
- 1 tbsp baking powder
- 1 tsp pumpkin pie spice
- ½ tsp salt
- 1 cup pumpkin puree
- ¾ cup low-fat milk, plus 2 tbsp
- 3 tbsp pure maple syrup
- 2 tbsp olive oil
- 1 tsp vanilla extract

DIRECTIONS

1. In a blender, add all ingredients and pulse until well combined.
2. Transfer the mixture into a bowl and set aside for about 10 minutes.
3. Heat a greased non-stick skillet over medium heat.
4. Place about ¼ cup of the mixture and spread in an even circle.
5. Cook for about 2 minutes per side.
6. Repeat with the remaining mixture.
7. Serve warm.

NUTRITION

- Calories: 113
- Carbs: 16.5 g
- Protein: 3.6 g
- Fat: 4.4 g
- Sugar: 5.9 g
- Sodium: 143 mg
- Fiber: 2 g

19. Sper-Tasty Chicken Muffins

Preparation time: 15 minutes
Cooking time: 45 minutes
Servings: 8

INGREDIENTS

- 8 eggs
- Salt and freshly ground black pepper, as required
- 2 tbsp filtered water
- 7 oz cooked chicken, chopped finely
- 1 ½ cup fresh spinach, chopped
- 1 cup green bell pepper, seeded and chopped finely
- 2 tbsp fresh parsley, chopped finely

NUTRITION

- Calories: 107
- Carbs: 1.7 g
- Protein: 13.1 g
- Fat: 5.2 g
- Sugar: 1.1 g
- Sodium: 102 mg
- Fiber: 0.4 g

DIRECTIONS

1. Preheat the oven to 350°F. Grease 8 cups of a muffin tin.
2. In a bowl, add eggs, salt, black pepper, and water and beat until well combined.
3. Add the chicken, spinach, bell pepper, and parsley and stir to combine.
4. Transfer the mixture into the prepared muffin cup evenly.
5. Bake for about 18–20 minutes or until golden brown.
6. Remove the muffin tin from the oven and place it onto a wire rack to cool for about 10 minutes.
7. Carefully invert the muffins onto a platter and serve warm.

---

20. Classic Zucchini Bread

Preparation time: 45 minutes
Cooking time: 15 minutes
Servings: 24

INGREDIENTS

- 3 cups all-purpose flour
- 2 tsp baking soda
- 1 tsp ground cinnamon
- 1 tsp ground nutmeg
- 2 cups Splenda
- 1 cup olive oil
- 3 eggs, beaten
- 2 tsp vanilla extract
- 2 cups zucchini, peeled, seeded, and grated

NUTRITION

- Calories: 219
- Carbs: 28.4 g
- Protein: 16.3 g
- Fat: 9.2 g
- Sugar: 16.3 g
- Sodium: 113 mg
- Fiber: 0.6 g

DIRECTIONS

1. Preheat the oven to 325°F. Arrange a rack in the center of the oven. Grease 2 loaf pans.
2. In a medium bowl, mix together the flour, baking soda, and spices.
3. In another large bowl, add the Splenda and oil and beat until well combined.
4. Add the eggs and vanilla extract and beat until well combined.
5. Add the flour mixture and mix until just combined.
6. Gently, fold in the zucchini.
7. Place the mixture into the bread loaf pans evenly.
8. Bake for about 45–50 minutes or until a toothpick inserted in the center of the bread comes out clean.
9. Remove the bread pans from the oven and place them onto a wire rack to cool for about 15 minutes.
10. Carefully, invert the bread onto the wire rack to cool completely before slicing
11. With a sharp knife, cut each bread loaf into desired-sized slices and serve.

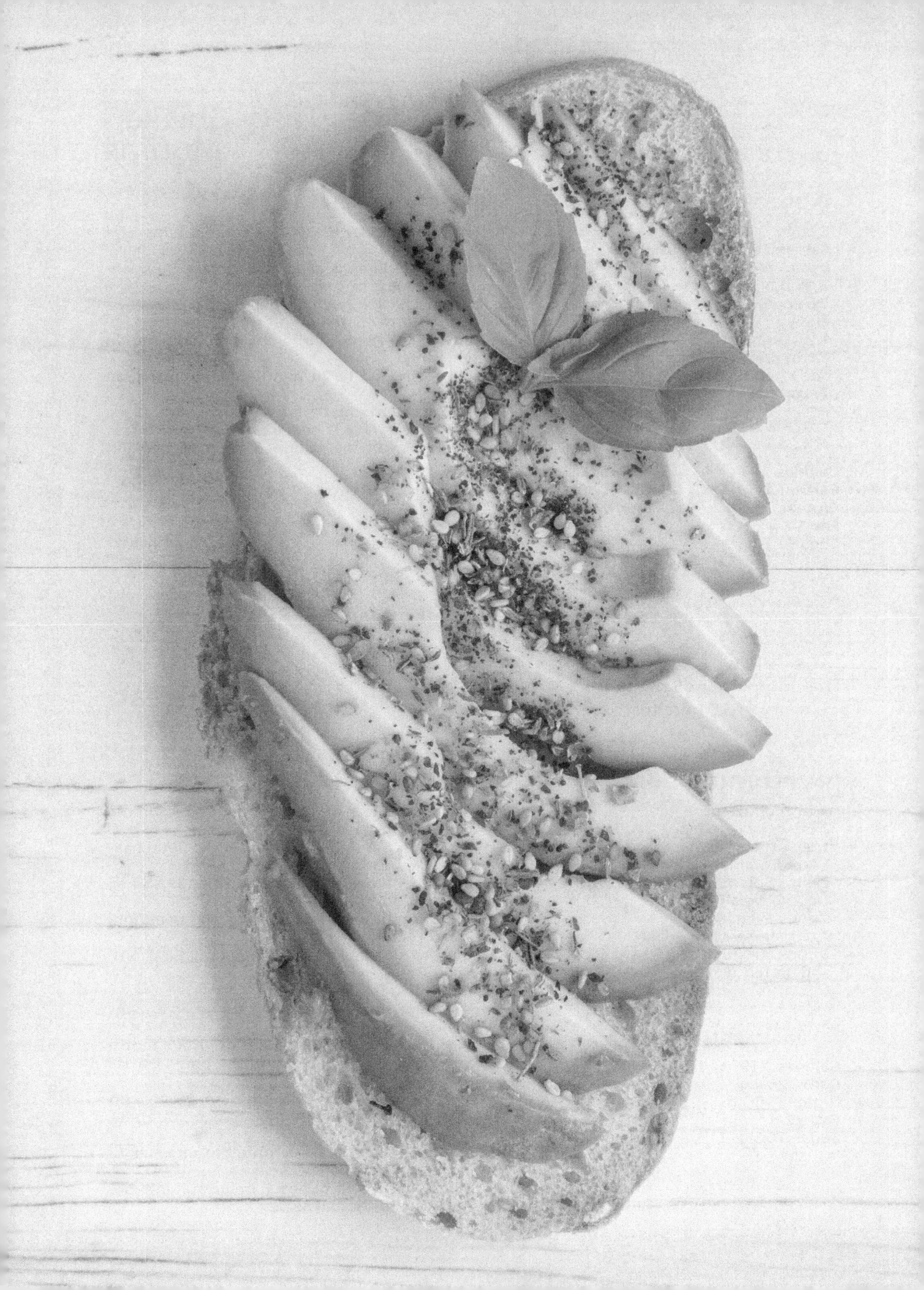

Chapter 6. High-Fiber Recipes

21. Pineapple Raspberry Parfaits

Preparation time: 5 minutes
Cooking time: 0 minutes
Servings: 4

INGREDIENTS

- 2 cups non-fat peach yogurt
- ½ pint raspberries
- 1 ½ cup pineapple chunks

DIRECTIONS

1. Place pineapple, raspberries, and yogurt into 4 glasses.
2. Serve and enjoy!

NUTRITION

- Calories: 155
- Carbs: 33 g
- Protein: 5.7 g
- Fat: 0.5 g
- Fiber: 2.9 g

22. Berry Chia Pudding

Preparation time: 5 minutes
Cooking time: 0 minutes
Chill time: 8 hours
Servings: 2

INGREDIENTS

- 1 ¾ cup blackberries, raspberries, or diced mango
- 1 cup unsweetened almond milk
- ¼ cup chia seeds
- 1 tbsp pure maple syrup
- ¾ tsp vanilla extract
- ½ cup whole-milk plain Greek yogurt
- ¼ cup granola

DIRECTIONS

1. Add milk and 1 ¼ cups fruit into the blender and blend until smooth.
2. Transfer it to the medium bowl. Add vanilla, syrup, and chia and combine well. Place it in the refrigerator for 8 hours.
3. Place pudding into the 2 bowls. Layering each serving with 2 tbsp granola, ¼ cup yogurt, and the remaining ¼ cup of fruit.
4. Serve!

NUTRITION

- Calories: 343
- Carbs: 39.4 g
- Protein: 13.8 g
- Fat: 15.4 g
- Fiber: 14.9 g

23. Spinach Avocado Smoothie

Preparation time: 5 minutes
Cooking time: 0 minutes
Servings: 1

INGREDIENTS

- 1 cup non-fat plain yogurt
- 1 cup fresh spinach
- 1 froz en banana
- ¼ avocado
- 2 tbsp water
- 1 tsp honey

DIRECTIONS

1. Mix the honey, water, avocado, banana, spinach, and yogurt into the blender and blend until smooth.
2. Serve and enjoy!

NUTRITION

- Calories: 357
- Carbs: 57.8 g
- Protein: 17.7 g
- Fat: 8.2 g
- Fiber: 7.8 g

---

24. Strawberry Pineapple Smoothie

Preparation time: 5 minutes
Cooking time: 0 minutes
Servings: 1

INGREDIENTS

- 1 cup froz en strawberries
- 1 cup chopped fresh pineapple
- ¾ cup chilled unsweetened almond milk
- 1 tbsp almond butter

DIRECTIONS

1. Mix the almond butter, almond milk, pineapple, and strawberries into the blender and process until smooth.
2. Add almond milk more if required.
3. Serve and enjoy!

NUTRITION

- Calories: 255
- Carbs: 39 g
- Protein: 5.6 g
- Fat: 11.1 g
- Fiber: 7.8 g

Preparation time: 10 minutes
Cooking time: 0 minutes
Servings: 2

25. Peach Blueberry Parfaits

INGREDIENTS

- 6 oz vanilla, peach, or blueberry fat-free yogurt
- 1 cup sweetener multigrain cluster cereal
- 1 peach, pitted and sliced
- ½ cup fresh blueberries
- ¼ tsp ground cinnamon

DIRECTIONS

1. Add half of the yogurt into the 2 glasses.
2. Top with half of the cereal. Top with half of cinnamon, blueberries, and peaches. Place the remaining blueberries, peaches, cereal, and yogurt.
3. Serve and enjoy!

NUTRITION

- Calories: 166
- Carbs: 34 g
- Protein: 11 g
- Fat: 1 g
- Fiber: 7 g

Preparation time: 5 minutes
Cooking time: 0 minutes
Servings: 1

26. Raspberry Yogurt Cereal Bowl

INGREDIENTS

- 1 cup non-fat plain yogurt
- ½ cup shredded wheat cereal
- ¼ cup fresh raspberries
- 2 tsp mini chocolate chips
- 1 tsp pumpkin seeds
- ¼ tsp ground cinnamon

DIRECTIONS

1. Add yogurt into the bowl.
2. Top with cinnamon, pumpkin seeds, chocolate chips, raspberries, and shredded wheat.
3. Serve and enjoy!

NUTRITION

- Calories: 290
- Carbs: 47.8 g
- Protein: 18.4 g
- Fat: 4.6 g
- Fiber: 6 g

27. Avocado Toast

Preparation time: 10 minutes
Cooking time: 2 minutes
Servings: 1

INGREDIENTS

- 1 cup mixed salad greens
- 1 tsp red-wine vinegar
- 1 tsp extra-virgin olive oil
- A pinch of salt
- A pinch of pepper
- 2 slices of sprouted whole-wheat bread, toasted
- ¼ cup plain hummus
- ¼ cup alfalfa sprouts
- ¼ sliced avocado
- 2 tsp unsalted sunflower seeds

DIRECTIONS

1. Firstly, toss greens with pepper, salt, oil, and vinegar into the bowl.
2. Spread each slice of toast with 2 tbsp hummus and top with greens, sprouts, avocado, and spinach.
3. Sprinkle with sunflower seeds.
4. Serve and enjoy!

NUTRITION

- Calories: 429
- Carbs: 46.4 g
- Protein: 16.2 g
- Fat: 21.9 g
- Fiber: 15.1 g

---

28. Loaded Pita Pockets

Preparation time: 5 minutes
Cooking time: 0 minutes
Servings: 1

INGREDIENTS

- 1 whole-wheat pita, halved
- ½ cup low-fat cottage cheese
- 4 chopped walnut halves
- 1 sliced banana

DIRECTIONS

1. Fill each pita with banana, walnuts, and cottage cheese.

NUTRITION

- Calories: 307
- Carbs: 46 g
- Protein: 21 g
- Fat: 8.5 g
- Fiber: 11 g

Lunch recipes

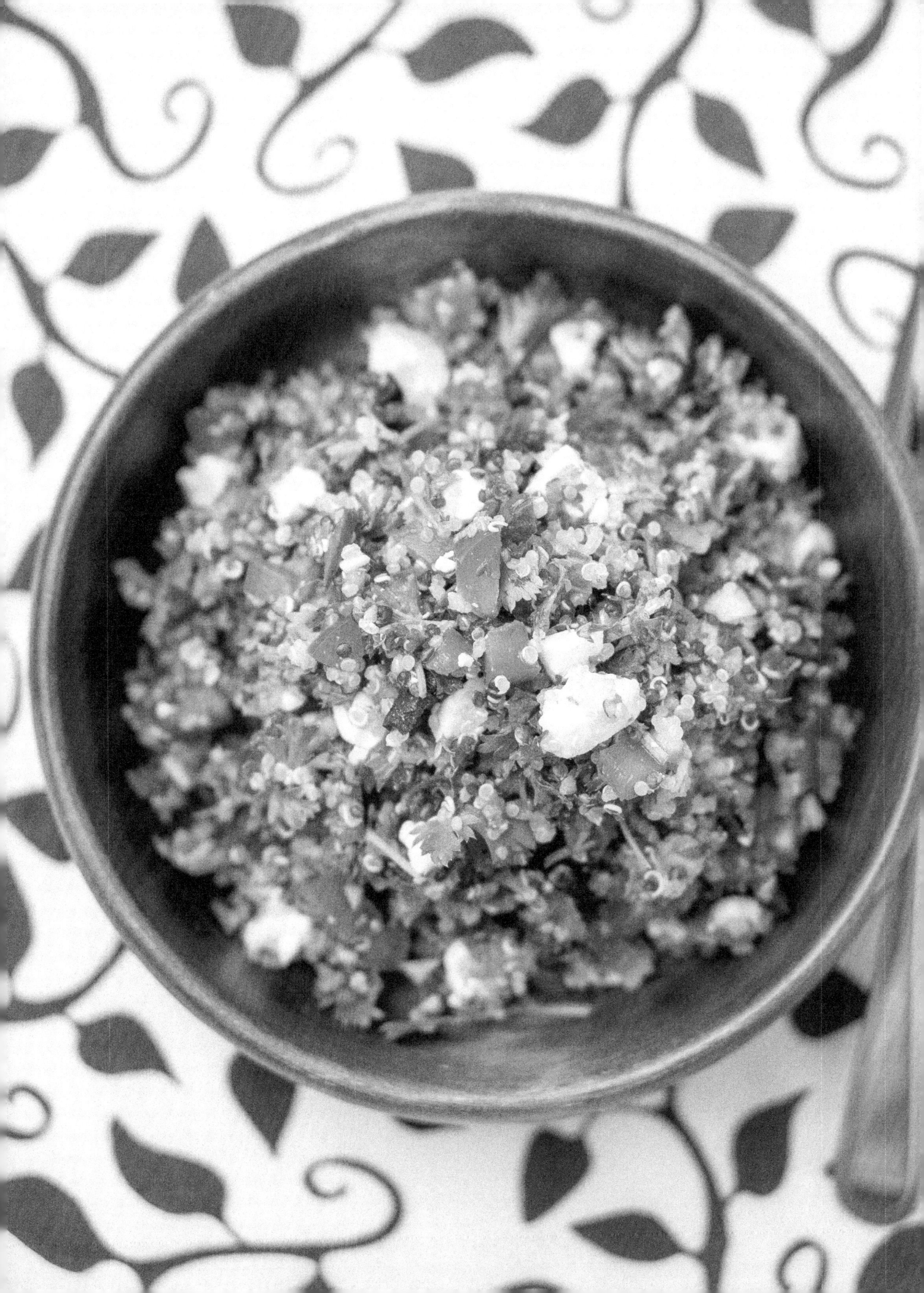

Chapter 7. Clear Liquid Recipes

Preparation time: 15 minutes
Cooking time: 10 minutes
Servings: 4

29. Grilled Vegetable Wrap Recipe with Hummus

INGREDIENTS
- 12 oz eggplant
- 1 large zucchini
- 1 red bell pepper
- 2 tbsp olive oil
- ½ tsp salt
- ½ tsp ground pepper
- ¾ tsp ground dried rosemary
- ¼ cup hummus
- 4 wholes wheat tortillas
- 6 large basil leaves, thinly sliced

DIRECTIONS
1. Preheat grill to medium-high temperature.
2. Using a 12-inch slicer, cut the eggplant into 1-inch slices (12 slices). Zoodles should be cut in half crosswise. Each half should be cut into 1-inch pieces (a total of 8 slices).
3. On a baking sheet, arrange the eggplant and zucchini slices. Season with salt and pepper and brush with olive oil on both sides.
4. Grill for 4 minutes on each side for eggplant and 3 minutes per side for zucchini and red bell pepper, or until the veggies are tender but not overdone.
5. Cut the veggies into strips and place them on a cutting board.
6. Distribute 1 tablespoon of mayonnaise on every whole-wheat tortilla, then divide the grilled veggies and basil leaves among the 4 wrap sandwiches.
7. Fold the tortilla in half from the bottom and then in half from the sides. Serve.

NUTRITION
- Calories: 231.6
- Protein: 5.7 g
- Carbs: 25.4 g
- Fat: 14.3 g

Preparation time: 10 minutes
Cooking time: 8 minutes
Servings: 4

30. Mediterranean Grilled Chicken Wrap

INGREDIENTS
- 1 ½ lb chicken tenders' Nature's Promise
- 1 tbsp olive oil
- 6 wholes wheat tortilla wraps Nature's Promise
- 8 oz container garlic hummus Nature's Promise, roasted
- 1 cup Baby spinach Nature's Promise
- 1 diced cucumber
- ¼ cup Grape tomatoes Nature's Promise, chopped
- ¼ cup Feta cheese, crumbled
- 1 tbsp Spice blend
- ½ tsp oregano
- ½ tsp paprika
- ¼ tsp cumin
- ¼ tsp sea salt
- ⅛ tsp garlic powder

DIRECTIONS
1. Preheat the grill to medium heat (350–400°F). Combine the spice mixture in a mixing bowl. Place the "chicken tenders" in a large mixing basin, drizzle with oil, and evenly coat with spices. Grill until the chicken is fully done.
2. On each tortilla wrap, spread a couple of tablespoons of hummus. Top each with a large handful of spinach and some chicken, then the cucumber, tomato, and Feta. To wrap, fold 1 side over the filling, then roll.

NUTRITION
- Calories: 551
- Protein: 34 g
- Carbs: 54 g
- Fat: 22 g

Preparation time: 10 minutes
Cooking time: 5 minutes
Servings: 4

31. Green Goodness Sandwich

INGREDIENTS

- 2 avocados ripe
- 1 tsp fresh lemon juice
- Salt and pepper to taste
- 1 cup Baby spinach
- ¼ cup goat cheese crumbled
- Freshly grounded pepper to taste
- 1 tbsp. Fresh chives, diced
- 1 Cucumber, thinly sliced
- 2 cups Sprouts, pea, sunflower, alfalfa, etc.
- 2 slices thick of grainy bread, toasted

DIRECTIONS

1. Cut the avocado in half, remove the pit, and scrape the contents into a small basin. Mash it with a fork till just a few chunks remain. Toss in the lemon juice and season with salt and pepper to taste.
2. Add a generous amount of (freshly ground) pepper to the crumbled goat cheese before serving
3. Toast the bread until it is golden brown. Once the slices are toasted, butter them and spread grainy/Dijon mustard on 1 slice of each sandwich. A layer of young spinach should be placed on top of the mustard. Place a layer of mashed avocado on top of the spinach. Serve the avocado with crumbled goat cheese over the top. Diced chives are put on top of the goat cheese. Add another layer of cucumber, then a covering of sprouts on top. Place the "top" slice of bread on top. To serve, push down slightly to compress and cut in half diagonally.

NUTRITION

- Calories: 397
- Protein: 9 g
- Carbs: 17 g
- Fat: 8 g

Preparation time: 10 minutes
Cooking time: 5 minutes
Servings: 5

32. Turkey, Brie, and Apple Sandwich with Apple Cider Mayo

INGREDIENTS

- 1 loaf of French bread sandwich, pre-sliced
- 3-4 Granny Smith apples
- 8 oz package of brie cheese, sliced into thin strips
- ½-pound turkey breast thick-cut, fresh from the deli counter
- 2 tbsp apple cider vinegar
- 6 tbsp mayonnaise
- 1 cup Arugula

DIRECTIONS

1. In a toaster, lightly toast your bread slices.
2. Set aside your granny apple after slicing them.
3. Combine the mayonnaise and apple cider vinegar in a small mixing bowl.
4. To make the sandwich, put about a tablespoon of mayo (somewhat depending on personal liking) on 1 slice of bread, then layer the brie, turkey, and apples on top. Finish with arugula and the top bread piece.

NUTRITION

- Calories: 556
- Protein: 26 g
- Carbs: 49 g
- Fat: 28 g

Preparation time: 10 minutes
Cooking time: 5 minutes
Servings: 5

33. Black Beans and Cauliflower Rice (Gluten-Free, Vegan/Plant-Based)

INGREDIENTS

- 1 can of about 15.5 oz black beans, rinsed and drained
- 1 large head cauliflower, 3 rounded cups riced
- 2 tbsp olive oil
- 3 fresh garlic cloves, minced
- ½ cup sweet onion, fresh and chopped
- ½ cup red bell pepper, fresh and diced
- ¼ tsp ground cayenne pepper for taste
- 3 tbsp jalapeno pickled slices, finely chopped
- Sea salt and black pepper to taste
- ½ cup diced fresh parsley (or cilantro)

DIRECTIONS

1. Black beans should be rinsed and drained. While prepping the veggies, set the vegetables on paper towels or a flat surface to absorb any residual water.
2. Take a thick core from the cauliflower and cut it into florets. To make "rice," pulse the ingredients in a food processor in tiny batches. Empty into a large mixing basin and repeat the process. Remove any uncut bits of the core and toss them out. Instead of using a food processor, a box grater may be utilized. About three full (rounded) cups of cauliflower "rice" are required. Remove from the equation.
3. In a medium/large skillet, preheat the olive oil over medium heat. Sauté the garlic in the olive oil until it turns golden. Stir in the bell pepper, onion, cayenne pepper, salt, and black pepper to the garlic and cook, turning periodically until the onion turns translucent. Stir in the pickled jalapeño. Pour cauliflower over veggies, season with salt n black pepper, and toss to combine. Cook for another 5–7 minutes, tossing and stirring halfway through (until cauliflower is tender but not mushy). Cook for a further 2 minutes after adding the black beans (enough to soften warm and gently beans). Add the parsley and combine thoroughly before serving

NUTRITION

- Calories: 398
- Protein: 18 g
- Carbs: 26 g
- Fat: 14 g

34. Avocado Sauce Pasta

Preparation time: 5 minutes
Cooking time: 10 minutes
Servings: 3

INGREDIENTS

- 2 cups uncooked dry pasta
- 1 ripe avocado halved, seeded and peeled
- ¼ cup olive oil
- ¼ cup grated Parmesan or Romano cheese
- ¼ cup fresh basil leaves
- 2 garlic cloves
- 2 tbsp lemon or lime juice
- Salt and freshly ground black pepper to taste

DIRECTIONS

1. Follow the package directions for cooking your pasta. Drain thoroughly.
2. In the blender or food processor, combine the avocados, olive oil, Parmesan cheese, cilantro, garlic, and lime juice, while the pasta is cooking You may either leave it thick or blend it till smooth.
3. Combine the spaghetti and the avocado sauce in a mixing bowl. Season to taste with salt and pepper, and if wanted, sprinkle with Parmesan and Romano cheese. Enjoy.

NUTRITION

- Calories: 37
- Protein: 0.5 g
- Carbs: 1.6 g
- Fat: 3.5 g

---

35. Greek Quinoa Bowls

Preparation time: 3 minutes
Cooking time: 12 minutes
Servings: 3

INGREDIENTS

- 1 cup quinoa
- 1 ½ cup water
- 1 cup green bell pepper, chopped
- 1 cup red bell pepper, chopped
- ⅓ cup Feta cheese, crumbled
- ¼ cup extra-virgin olive oil
- 2-3 tbs papple cider vinegar
- Salt and pepper to taste
- 1-2 tbsp fresh parsley

Extras:
- Hummus
- Pita wedges
- Olives
- Fresh tomatoes
- Sliced or chopped avocado
- Lemon wedges

DIRECTIONS

1. Using the mesh strainer or sieve, rinse and drain your quinoa.
2. Briefly toast quinoa in a medium saucepan over medium heat to drain any excess water. For a few minutes, stir while it toasts. This step is optional, although it enhances the quinoa's nuttiness and fluff factor.
3. After that, add your water, increase the heat to high, and bring to a boil.
4. Reduce heat to low and cook for 12–13 minutes, or until quinoa is frothy and liquid has been absorbed, covered with a little ajar lid.
5. While the quinoa is cooking, cut and prepare the additional ingredients, and mix the ingredients for the dressing
6. Take the now-fluffy quinoa out of the saucepan and puff it up with a fork.
7. You may chill the quinoa for a few minutes before adding your veggies to make a chilled salad, or just let it rest on the counter for a few minutes to make a room temp quinoa bowl. It's entirely up to you.
8. Whisk together apple cider vinegar, olive oil, salt, and pepper to make the vinaigrette. How simple was that? Pour over quinoa dish and mix with forks/salad servers before digging in.
9. If preferred, season with more salt and pepper to taste.

NUTRITION

- Calories: 468
- Protein: 17 g
- Carbs: 58 g
- Fat: 19 g

Preparation time: 5 minutes
Cooking time: 10 minutes
Servings: 3

36. Baked Sweet Potato Tacos

INGREDIENTS

- 2 medium sweet potatoes
- 1 tsp black beans
- 1 tsp cumin
- 1 tsp chili powder
- ¼ cup green onion, chopped
- 1 tsp lime juice
- Chopped tomatoes, sliced avocado, salsa, hot sauce, or any other desired toppings

DIRECTIONS

1. Potatoes should be washed and pierced with a fork.
2. Microwave it for 8–10 minutes, or till cooked through, wrapped in a moist paper towel.
3. Allow cooling slightly before cutting each potato in half and scooping out the meat while keeping the skin intact. Remove from the equation.
4. Heat black beans, sweet potato, chili powder, cumin, and lime juice in a small skillet over medium heat until cooked through, about 5 minutes.
5. Fill sweet potato skins with sweet potato mixture.
6. Serve with chosen toppings on top.

NUTRITION

- Calories: 405
- Protein: 11 g
- Carbs: 53 g
- Fat: 17 g

Preparation time: 10 minutes
Cooking time: 45 minutes
Servings: 6

37. 5-Ingredient Sweet Potato Black Bean Chili

INGREDIENTS

- 1 medium diced white or yellow onion
- 3 medium sweet potatoes
- 1 (16 oz) jar of salsa (chunky is preferred)
- 1 (15 oz) can of black beans (with salt)
- 2 cups vegetable stock
- 2 cups water

Optional spices:
- 1 tbsp chili powder
- 2 tsp ground cumin
- ½ tsp ground cinnamon
- ½ tsp chipotle powder
- 1–2 tsp hot sauce

For Servings:
- Fresh cilantro
- Chopped red onion
- Guac or avocado
- Lime juice

DIRECTIONS

1. Sweat onions in 1 tbsp oil in a big saucepan over medium heat, seasoning with a good dose of salt and pepper (amounts as indicated, use if changing batch size). Cook, occasionally stirring, over medium heat until the vegetables are transparent and tender.
2. At this point, add the sweet potato and any seasonings you choose. 3 minutes in the oven. After that, mix in the salsa, water, and vegetable stock.
3. On medium-high heat, bring the mixture to a low boil, then reduce to medium-low and continue to cook. Cook for a further 20 minutes, ideally 30 minutes, or till the "sweet potatoes" are fork-tender and the soup has thickened. This soup tastes best if you make it the night before or let it sit for several hours so the flavors can mingle with the veggies and beans.
4. Fresh cilantro, avocado, onion, and lime juice can be added to the dish. Chips work well as a spoon.

NUTRITION

- Calories: 213
- Protein: 6 g
- Carbs: 47 g
- Fat: 0.6 g

Preparation time: 15 minutes
Cooking time: 15 minutes
Servings: 6

38. Whole-Wheat Pasta with Fresh Tomatoes and Herbs

INGREDIENTS

- ½ lb (cut into ½-inch pieces) ripe tomatoes fresh, cored
- 3 tbsp fresh basil, minced
- 1 tbsp minced fresh oregano
- 1 garlic clove, minced
- ¼ cup olive oil
- Salt and pepper to taste
- 1 lb whole-wheat pasta

DIRECTIONS

1. In a medium mixing bowl, combine the tomatoes, herbs, garlic, and oil. To taste, season with salt and freshly ground pepper. Remove from the equation.
2. In a big saucepan, bring water to a boil. 1 tbsp salt + 1 tbsp water. Cook the pasta according to the package recommendations for al dente. 1-2 cups of pasta boiling water should be set aside. Return the spaghetti to the saucepan after draining it. Toss in the tomato sauce and mix well. If the sauce needs to be thinned, add a few of the pasta water.

NUTRITION

- Calories: 366
- Protein: 12 g
- Carbs: 10 g
- Fat: 0.8 g

Preparation time: 5 minutes
Cooking time: 10 minutes
Servings: 4

39. Honey Mustard Salmon with Shaved Brussel Sprout Salad

INGREDIENTS

- 4 salmon filets
- 2 tbsp honey
- 2 tbsp Dijon mustard
- Juice of small lemon
- Salt and pepper to taste

For the salad:
- 16 oz Brussel sprouts (shaved)
- 1 small Fuji apple sliced thin
- 2 tbsp rice wine vinegar
- 1 tsp honey

DIRECTIONS

1. Preheat the oven to broil. Combine honey, lemon juice, and Dijon mustard in a small bowl for salmon fillets. Coat all fillets in the batter and broil for 5 minutes, or till cooked through and lightly browned.
2. Combine rice wine vinegar and honey in a separate small bowl. Toss the Brussel sprouts and apples together.
3. Allow the salmon to chill before adding it to the Brussel sprout salad.

NUTRITION

- Calories: 110
- Protein: 1 g
- Carbs: 2 g
- Fat: 0.5 g

Preparation time: 5 minutes
Cooking time: 5 minutes
Servings: 4

40. 5-Minute Tomato Salad Lentil

INGREDIENTS

- 15 oz can of lentils (1 ½ cups cooked)
- 1 ½ cups cherry tomatoes
- ¼ cup white wine vinegar (or the white balsamic vinegar)
- ⅛ cup chives (optional)
- Salt for taste
- Optional: olive oil, parsley, basil, etc.

DIRECTIONS

1. Lentils should be rinsed and drained. Cherry tomatoes should be quartered or halved. Chop the chives.
2. Toss all of the ingredients together in a small mixing dish. Season to taste with salt and vinegar, if needed.
3. Serve right away or keep refrigerated in an airtight container to let flavors meld.

NUTRITION

- Calories: 137
- Protein: 10 g
- Carbs: 24 g
- Fat: 1 g

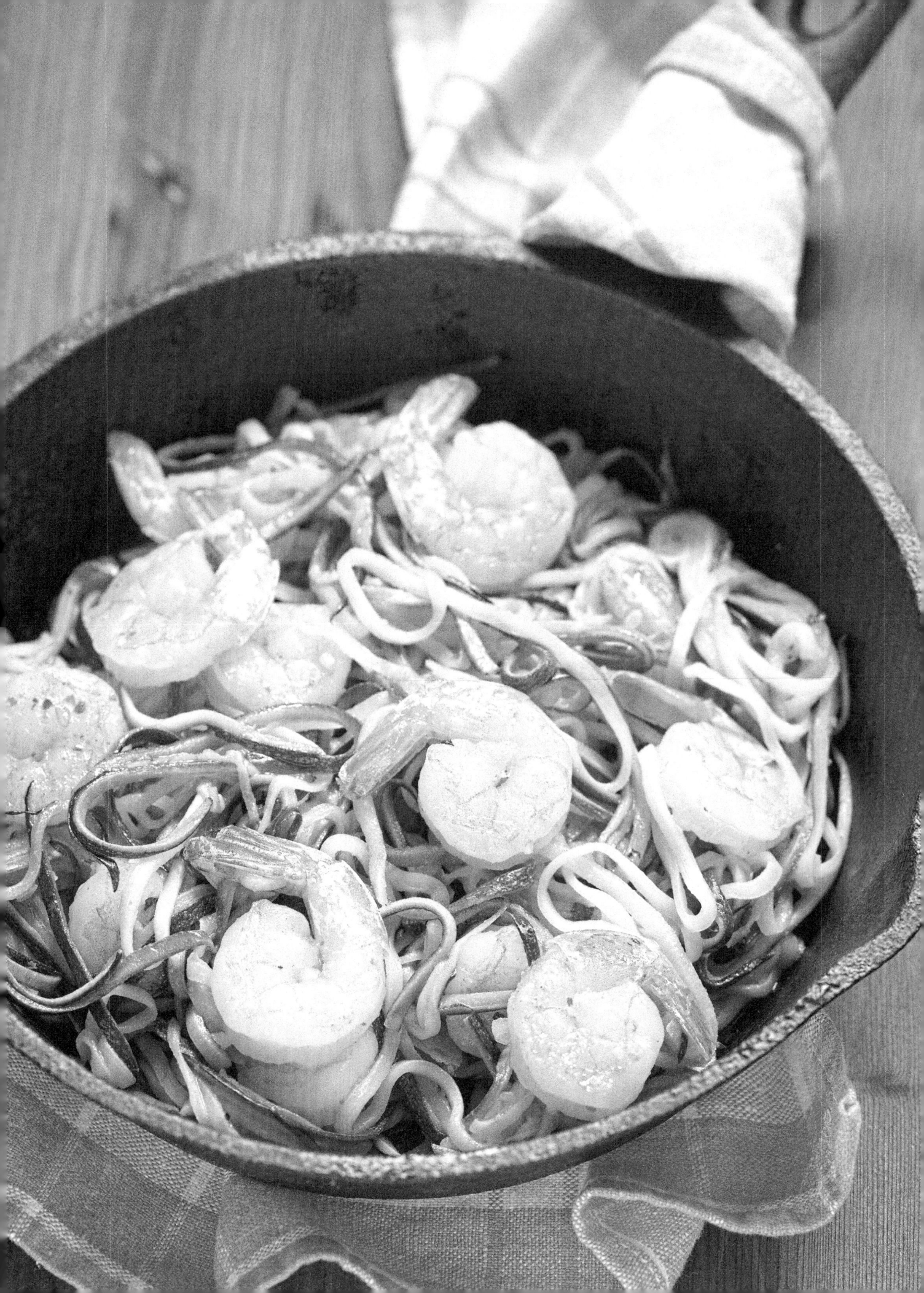

Chapter 8. Low-Residue Recipes

Preparation time: 30 minutes
Cooking time: 16 minutes
Servings: 4

41. Veggies and Apple with Orange Sauce

INGREDIENTS

For the sauce:

- 1 (1-inch) fresh ginger, minced
- 2 garlic cloves, minced
- 1 tbsp fresh orange zest, grated finely
- ½ cup fresh orange juice
- 2 tbsp white wine vinegar
- 2 tbsp coconut aminos
- 1 tbsp red boat fish sauce

For the veggies and apple:

- 1 tbsp extra-virgin olive oil
- 1 cup carrot, peeled and julienned
- 1 cup celery, chopped
- 1 cup onion, chopped
- 2 apples, cored and sliced

DIRECTIONS

1. In a sizable bowl, mix all sauce ingredients. Keep aside.
2. In a big skillet, set the oil on medium-high heat.
3. Add the carrot and stir fry for about 4–5 minutes.
4. Attach celery and onion. Stir fry for approximately 4–5 minutes.
5. Pour the sauce and stir to combine. Cook for approximately 2–3 minutes.
6. Stir in apple slices and cook for about 2–3 minutes more.
7. Serve hot.

NUTRITION

- Calories: 29
- Fat: 1 g
- Carbs: 2 g
- Fiber: 1 g
- Protein: 1 g

Preparation time: 15 minutes
Cooking time: 21 minutes
Servings: 4

42. Cauliflower Rice with Prawns and Veggies

INGREDIENTS

- 2 tbsp coconut oil, divided
- 14 prawns, peeled and deveined
- 2 organic eggs, beaten
- 1 brown onion, chopped
- 1 garlic clove, minced
- 1 small fresh red chili, chopped
- ½ lb grass-fed ground chicken
- 1 cauliflower head, cut into florets, processed like rice consistency
- ¼ red cabbage, chopped
- ½ cup green peas, shelled
- 1 head small broccoli
- 1 large carrot, peeled and finely chopped
- 1 small red bell pepper
- 2 bok choy, sliced thinly
- 3 tbsp coconut aminos
- Salt and freshly ground black pepper

DIRECTIONS

1. In a substantial skillet, heat ½ tablespoon of oil on medium-high heat.
2. Add the prawns and cook for approximately 3-4 minutes. Transfer to a large bowl.
3. In the same skillet, heat ½ tablespoon of oil on medium heat.
4. Add the beaten eggs and with the back of a spoon, spread the eggs. Cook for around 2 minutes.
5. Remove the eggs from the skillet and cut them into strips.
6. In the identical skillet, heat the remaining oil on high heat. Add the onion, garlic, and red chili. Sauté for about 4-5 minutes.
7. Add the chicken and cook for about 4-5 minutes.
8. Add the cauliflower rice and remaining veggies except for the bok choy and coconut aminos and cook for around 2-3 minutes.
9. Add the bok choy, coconut aminos, cooked eggs, prawns, salt, and black pepper. Cook for 2 minutes more.

NUTRITION

- Calories: 75
- Carbs: 0.1 g
- Protein: 13.4 g
- Fat: 1.7 g
- Sugar: 0 g
- Sodium: 253 mg

Preparation time: 15 minutes
Cooking time: 10 minutes
Servings: 2

43. Lentils with Tomatoes and Turmeric

INGREDIENTS

- ½ onion, finely chopped
- ½ tsp garlic powder
- ½ (14 oz) can of chopped tomatoes, drained
- ⅛ tsp ground black pepper
- 1 tbsp extra-virgin olive oil, plus extra for garnishing
- ½ tbsp ground turmeric
- ½ (14 oz) can lentils, drained
- ¼ tsp sea salt

DIRECTIONS

1. Heat the olive oil in a pot over medium-high heat until it starts shimmering
2. Cook, stirring regularly, for around 5 minutes until the onion and turmeric are tender.
3. Add the garlic powder, salt, tomatoes, lentils, and pepper.
4. Cook, stirring regularly, for 5 minutes

NUTRITION

- Calories: 248
- Fat: 8 g
- Carbs: 34 g
- Sugar: 5 g
- Fiber: 15 g
- Protein: 12 g
- Sodium: 243 mg

Preparation time: 10 minutes
Cooking time: 12 minutes
Servings: 2

44. Fried Rice with Kale

INGREDIENTS

- 4 oz tofu chopped
- 1 cup kale, stemmed and chopped
- 2 tbsp stir-fry sauce
- 1 tbsp extra-virgin olive oil
- 3 sliced scallions
- 1 ½ cup cooked brown rice

DIRECTIONS

1. Heat the olive oil in a big skillet or pan over medium-high heat until it starts shimmering
2. Add the scallions, tofu, and kale. Cook until the vegetables are tender.
3. Combine the stir-fry sauce and brown rice in a mixing bowl. Cook, stirring regularly until thoroughly heated.

NUTRITION

- Calories: 301
- Fat: 11 g
- Carbs: 36 g
- Sugar: 1 g
- Fiber: 3 g
- Protein: 16 g
- Sodium: 2.535 mg

Preparation time: 10 minutes
Cooking time: 12 minutes
Servings: 2

45. Stir-Fry Tofu and Red Pepper

INGREDIENTS

- 1 chopped red bell peppers
- 1 tbsp extra-virgin olive oil
- ½ chopped onion
- ¼ cup ginger teriyaki sauce
- 4 oz chopped tofu

DIRECTIONS

1. Heat the olive oil in a skillet or pan over medium-high heat until it starts shimmering
2. Add the onion, red bell peppers, and tofu. Cook, stirring regularly.
3. Apply the teriyaki sauce to the skillet or pan after whisking it together. Cook, stirring occasionally for 3–4 minutes, or until it thickens.

NUTRITION

- Calories: 166
- Fat: 10 g
- Carbs: 17 g
- Sugar: 12 g
- Fiber: 2 g
- Protein: 7 g
- Sodium: 892 mg

Preparation time: 10 minutes
Cooking time: 25 minutes
Servings: 2

46. Sweet Potato and Bell Pepper Hash with a Fried Egg

INGREDIENTS

- ½ chopped onion
- 2 cups peeled and cubed potatoes
- 2 tbsp extra-virgin olive oil
- ½ chopped red bell pepper
- ½ tsp sea salt
- 2 eggs
- A pinch of freshly ground black pepper

DIRECTIONS

1. Heat olive oil in a big non-stick pan over medium-high heat until it starts shimmering
2. Add the red bell pepper, onion, and sweet potato. Season with salt and a pinch of black pepper. Cook, stirring regularly until the potatoes are soft and browned.
3. Serve the potatoes in 4 bowls.
4. Return the skillet or pan to heat, turn the heat down to medium-low, and swirl to secure the bottom of the pan with the remaining olive oil.
5. Scatter some salt over the eggs and carefully smash them into the tray. Cook until the whites are set, around 3–4 minutes.
6. Flip the eggs gently and remove them from the heat. Allow to rest for 1 minute in the hot skillet or pan. 1 egg should be placed on top of each serving of hash.

NUTRITION

- Calories: 384
- Fat: 19 g
- Carbs: 47 g
- Sugar: 16 g
- Fiber: 8 g
- Protein: 10 g
- Sodium: 603 mg

Preparation time: 5 minutes
Cooking time: 25 minutes
Servings: 2

47. Quinoa Florentine

INGREDIENTS

- ½ chopped onion
- 2 minced garlic cloves
- 2 cups no-salt-added vegetable broth
- A pinch of freshly ground black pepper
- 1 tbsp extra-virgin olive oil
- 1 ½ cup fresh baby spinach
- 1 cup quinoa, rinsed well
- ¼ tsp sea salt

DIRECTIONS

1. Heat the olive oil over medium-high heat until it starts shimmering
2. Add the spinach and onion. Cook, stirring regularly, for 3 minutes.
3. Cook, stirring continuously, for 30 seconds after adding the garlic.
4. Combine the vegetable broth, salt, quinoa, and pepper in a mixing bowl. Set to a simmer, then reduce to low heat. Cook, covered, for 15–20 minutes, or until the liquid has been absorbed. Using a fork, fluff the mixture.

NUTRITION

- Calories: 403
- Fat: 12 g
- Carbs: 62 g
- Sugar: 4 g
- Fiber: 7 g
- Protein: 13 g
- Sodium: 278 mg

Preparation time: 5 minutes
Cooking time: 20 minutes
Servings: 2

48. Tomato Asparagus Frittata

INGREDIENTS

- 5 trimmed asparagus spears
- 3 eggs
- 1 tbsp extra-virgin olive oil
- 5 cherry tomatoes
- ½ tbsp chopped fresh thyme
- A pinch of freshly ground black pepper
- ¼ tsp sea salt

NUTRITION

- Calories: 224
- Fat: 14 g
- Carbs: 15 g
- Sugar: 10 g
- Fiber: 5 g
- Protein: 12 g
- Sodium: 343 mg

DIRECTIONS

1. Preheat the broiler to the highest setting
2. Heat the olive oil in a big ovenproof skillet or pan over medium-high heat until it starts shimmering
3. Toss in the asparagus. Cook, stirring regularly, for 5 minutes.
4. Add in the tomatoes. Cook for 3 minutes, stirring once in a while.
5. Whisk together the thyme, salt, eggs, and pepper in a medium mixing cup. Carefully, spill over the tomatoes and asparagus, turning them about in the pan to ensure that they are equally distributed.
6. Turn the heat down to medium. Cook for 3 minutes, or until the eggs are hardened around the outside
7. Place the pan under the broiler and cook for 3–5 minutes, or until puffed and brown. To eat, cut into wedges.

Preparation time: 15 minutes
Cooking time: 3 minutes
Servings: 6

49. Shrimp and Mango Salsa Lettuce Wraps

INGREDIENTS

For the salsa:
- 1 mango, peeled, pitted, and chopped
- ¼ cup red onion, finely chopped
- ½ cup red bell pepper
- ¼ cup fresh cilantro, chopped
- 1 jalapeño pepper, seeded and finely chopped
- 2 tbsp fresh lime juice
- Salt and freshly ground black pepper

For the shrimp wraps:
- 1 teaspoon organic olive oil
- 2 lb large shrimp, peeled, deveined, and chopped
- ½ teaspoon ground cumin
- 1 tbsp red chili powder
- Salt and freshly ground black pepper
- 2 heads of butter lettuce, leaves separated

DIRECTIONS

For the salsa:

1. In a large bowl, mix all ingredients. Keep aside.

For the shrimp wraps:

1. In a skillet, heat oil on medium heat.
2. Add the shrimp and seasoning Cook for approximately 2–3 minutes.
3. Remove from the heat and cool slightly.
4. Divide the shrimp mixture over lettuce leaves lightly.
5. Top with mango salsa evenly and serve.

NUTRITION

- Calories: 463
- Fat: 4 g
- Carbs: 75 g
- Fiber: 18 g
- Protein: 34 g

Preparation time: 25 minutes
Cooking time: 30 minutes
Servings: 6

50. Bacon-Wrapped Asparagus

INGREDIENTS

- 10 bacon slices cut in half
- 1 pound fresh asparagus, trimmed
- 1 tbsp extra-virgin olive oil
- 1 tbsp balsamic vinegar
- Freshly ground black pepper, to taste
- 1 lemon, sliced

DIRECTIONS

1. Heat the oven to 400°F. Line a substantial baking dish with foil paper.
2. Wrap 1 bacon slice around each asparagus piece.
3. Arrange asparagus in the prepared baking dish.
4. Set with oil and vinegar. Sprinkle with black pepper.
5. Bake for approximately 15 minutes. Change the inside and bake for 10-15 minutes more.
6. Serve immediately with lemon slices.

NUTRITION

- Calories: 645
- Fat: 32 g
- Carbs: 65 g
- Fiber: 5 g
- Protein: 26 g

Preparation time: 15 minutes
Cooking time: 21 minutes
Servings: 4

51. Zucchini Pasta with Shrimp

INGREDIENTS

- 2 tbsp ghee or coconut oil
- 1 tbsp extra-virgin olive oil
- 3 garlic cloves, minced
- 1 lb shrimp, peeled and deveined
- 4 large zucchinis, spiralized
- Salt and freshly ground black pepper
- 4-6 fresh basil leaves, chopped

DIRECTIONS

1. In a big skillet, heat the ghee and essential olive oil on medium heat.
2. Add garlic and sauté for approximately 1 minute.
3. Set the shrimp and cook for approximately 2-3 minutes.
4. Add the zucchini, tossing occasionally, and cook for approximately 2-3 minutes.
5. Stir in salt and black pepper and take off the heat.
6. Serve while using the garnishing of basil leaves.

NUTRITION

- Calories: 59
- Fat: 1 g
- Carbs: 14 g
- Fiber: 1 g
- Protein: 1 g
- Sodium: 304 mg

Preparation time: 25 minutes
Cooking time: 25 minutes
Servings: 1

52. Sweet Potato Buns Sandwich

INGREDIENTS

For the sweet potato buns:
- 1 ½ tbsp extra-virgin olive oil, divided
- 1 large sweet potato, peeled and spiralized
- 2 tsp garlic powder
- Salt and freshly ground black pepper
- 1 large organic egg
- 1 organic egg white

For the sandwich:
- 1 (½ oz) salmon piece
- Salt and freshly ground black pepper
- 1 tsp fresh lime juice
- 1 tomato, sliced
- 1 onion, sliced
- ½ avocado, peeled, pitted, and chopped
- 2 tsp fresh cilantro, chopped
- 1 large bit of fresh kale
- 1 bacon piece

NUTRITION

- Calories: 75
- Carbs: 0.1 g
- Protein: 13.4 g
- Fat: 1.7 g
- Sugar: 0 g
- Sodium: 253 mg

DIRECTIONS

For the buns:
1. In a sizable skillet, heat ½ tablespoon of oil on medium heat.
2. Add the sweet potato and sprinkle with garlic powder, salt, and black pepper.
3. Cook for 5–7 minutes. Transfer the sweet potato mixture to a bowl.
4. Add the egg and egg white; mix well. Now, transfer a combination into 2 (6 oz) ramekins, midway full.
5. Cover the ramekins with wax paper. Now, place them over noodles to press firmly down. Refrigerate for about 15–20 minutes.

For the sandwich:
1. Preheat the grill to medium heat. Grease it.
2. In another bowl, add salmon, salt, black pepper, and lime juice. Toss to coat well.
3. In a substantial skillet, heat the remaining oil on medium-low heat.
4. Carefully, transfer the sweet potato patties to the skillet.
5. Cook for 3–4 minutes. Change the medial side and cook for 2–3 minutes more.
6. Place the salmon, onion, and tomato slices over the grill.
7. Grill the tomato slice for 1 minute. Grate the onion slice for approximately 2 minutes.
8. Cook the salmon for approximately 4–5 minutes or till the desired doneness.
9. In a bowl, add the avocado and cilantro; mash well.
10. On a plate, place the onion slice, salmon, tomato, bacon, and kale over the bun.
11. Spread the avocado mash around the bottom side of another bun. Place the bun, and avocado mash side downwards over the kale.
12. Secure having a toothpick and serve.

53. Shrimp, Sausage, and Veggie Skillet

Preparation time: 15 minutes
Cooking time: 13 minutes
Servings: 3

INGREDIENTS

- 3 tbsp organic olive oil, divided
- 1 lb shrimp, peeled and deveined
- ½ medium yellow onion, chopped
- ¾ cup green peppers, seeded and chopped
- ¾ cup green peppers, seeded and chopped
- 1 zucchini, chopped
- 6 oz cooked sausage, chopped
- 2 garlic cloves, minced
- ¼ cup chicken broth
- A pinch of red pepper flakes, crushed
- Salt and freshly ground black pepper

DIRECTIONS

1. In a sizable skillet, heat 1 tablespoon of oil on medium-high heat.
2. Attach the shrimp and cook for around 3–4 minutes. Transfer it to a bowl.
3. In the same skillet, heat the remaining oil on medium heat.
4. Add the onion and sweet peppers. Sauté for about 4–5 minutes.
5. Stir in the zucchini and sausage. Cook for approximately 2 minutes.
6. Add the garlic and cooled shrimp. Cook for approximately 1 minute.
7. Pour the broth and mix to combine well. Stir in red pepper flakes, salt, and black pepper. Cook for approximately 1 minute.
8. Serve hot.

NUTRITION

- Calories: 332
- Fat: 18 g
- Carbs: 32 g
- Fiber: 9 g
- Protein: 12 g

---

54. Sea Scallops with Spinach and Bacon

Preparation time: 25 minutes
Cooking time: 25 minutes
Servings: 4

INGREDIENTS

- 3 bacon slices
- 1 ½ lb jumbo sea scallops
- Salt and freshly ground black pepper
- 1 cup onion, chopped
- 6 garlic cloves, minced
- 12 oz fresh baby spinach

DIRECTIONS

1. Heat a sizable non-stick skillet on medium-high heat.
2. Add the bacon and cook for approximately 8–10 minutes.
3. Transfer the bacon into a bowl, reserving 1 tablespoon of bacon fat within the skillet.
4. Chop the bacon and keep it aside.
5. Attach the scallops and sprinkle with salt and black pepper.
6. Immediately, boost the heat to high heat.
7. Cook for about 5 minutes, turning once after 2 ½ minutes.
8. Transfer the scallops into another bowl. Cover having foil paper to ensure that they're warm.
9. In the same skillet, add the onion and garlic minimizing the temperature to medium-high.
10. Sauté them for around 3 minutes.
11. Add the spinach and cook for approximately 2–3 minutes. Season with salt and black pepper. Remove from the heat.
12. Divide the spinach among serving plates. Top with scallops and bacon evenly. Serve immediately.

NUTRITION

- Calories: 246
- Fat: 13 g
- Carbs: 11 g
- Fiber: 1 g
- Protein: 22 g

Preparation time: 10 minutes
Cooking time: 26 minutes
Servings: 4

55. Liver with Onion and Parsley One

INGREDIENTS

- 3 tbsp coconut oil, divided
- 2 large onions, sliced
- Salt to taste
- 1 lb grass-fed beef liver, cut into ½-inch-thick slices
- Freshly ground black pepper, to taste
- ½ cup fresh parsley
- 2 tbsp freshly squeezed lemon juice

DIRECTIONS

1. In a sizable skillet, heat 1 tablespoon of oil on high heat.
2. Attach the onions plus some salt and sauté for about 5 minutes.
3. Set the heat to medium. Sauté them for 10–15 minutes more.
4. Place the onion right into a plate.
5. In the same skillet, heat another 1 tablespoon of oil on medium-high heat.
6. Add the liver and sprinkle with salt and black pepper.
7. Cook for approximately 1–2 minutes or till browned.
8. Flip alongside it and cook for approximately 1–2 minutes till browned. Set the liver right into a plate.
9. In the skillet, heat the remaining oil on medium heat.
10. Attach the cooked onion, parsley, and lemon juice; stir well. Cook for about 2–3 minutes.
11. Set the onion mixture over the liver and serve immediately.

NUTRITION

- Calories: 228
- Fat: 3 g
- Carbs: 43 g
- Fiber: 6 g
- Protein: 12 g

Preparation time: 10 minutes
Cooking time: 26 minutes
Servings: 5

56. Egg and Avocado Wraps

INGREDIENTS

- 1 ripe avocado, peeled, pitted, and chopped
- 1 tbsp freshly squeezed lemon juice
- 1 tbsp fresh parsley, chopped
- 2 tbsp celery stalk, chopped
- 4 organic hard-boiled eggs, peeled and finely chopped
- Salt and freshly ground black pepper
- 4–5 endive bulb s
- 2 cooked bacon slices, chopped

DIRECTIONS

1. In a bowl, add the avocado and freshly squeezed lemon juice and mash till smooth and creamy.
2. Add parsley, celery, eggs, salt, and black pepper. Stir to mix well.
3. Separate the endive leaves. Divide the avocado mixture over endive leaves evenly.
4. Top with bacon and serve immediately.

NUTRITION

- Calories: 404
- Fat: 7 g
- Carbs: 47 g
- Fiber: 6 g
- Protein: 15 g

Preparation time: 10 minutes
Cooking time: 28 minutes
Servings: 4

57. Creamy Sweet Potato Pasta with Pancetta

INGREDIENTS

For the creamy sauce:
- 4-5 cups cauliflower florets
- 1 small shallot, minced
- 1 large garlic herb, chopped
- A pinch of red pepper flakes, crushed
- 1 cup chicken broth
- 1 tbsp nutritional yeast
- Salt to taste

For the pancetta:
- 8 pancetta slices, cubed

For the sweet potato pasta:
- 1 tbsp extra-virgin olive oil
- 3 medium sweet potatoes, peeled and spiralized
- 3 cups leeks
- Salt and freshly ground black pepper
- 1 tbsp fresh parsley, chopped

DIRECTIONS

1. In a pan of salted boiling water, attach cauliflower florets and cook for around 7–8 minutes. Drain well.
2. Meanwhile, heat a large non-stick skillet on medium heat.
3. Add pancetta slices and cook for approximately 5–7 minutes.
4. Transfer the pancetta into a bowl.
5. In the same skillet, add shallot, garlic, and red pepper flakes. Sauté for around 2 minutes.
6. Transfer the shallot mixture into a higher speed blender.
7. Add the cauliflower and the remaining sauce ingredients. Pulse till smooth and creamy.
8. In the identical skillet, heat extra-virgin olive oil on medium heat.
9. Add sweet potatoes and leeks. Cook, tossing occasionally for approximately 8–10 minutes.
10. Stir in the sauce and cook for about 1 minute.
11. Serve this creamy pasta with all the topping of the pancetta and parsley.

NUTRITION

- Calories: 33
- Carbs: 8.1 g
- Protein: 0.2 g
- Fat: 0.1 g
- Sugar: 7.6 g
- Sodium: 130 mg
- Fiber: 0.1 g

Preparation time: 10 minutes
Cooking time: 15 minutes
Servings: 3

58. Roasted Beet Pasta with Kale and Pesto

INGREDIENTS

For the pesto:
- 3 cups fresh basil leaves
- 1 large garlic oil
- ¼ cup organic olive oil
- ¼ cup pine nuts
- Salt and freshly ground black pepper

For the beet pasta:
- 2 medium beets, trimmed, peeled, and spiralized
- Olive oil cooking spray, as required
- Salt and freshly ground black pepper

For the kale:
- 2 cups fresh baby kale

DIRECTIONS

1. Heat the oven to 425°F. Lightly, grease a large baking sheet.
2. In a mixer, add all pesto ingredients and pulse till smooth. Keep aside.
3. Place the beet pasta on the prepared baking sheet.
4. Drizzle with cooking spray and sprinkle with salt and black pepper. Gently, toss to coat well.
5. Roast for around 5-10 minutes or till the desired doneness.
6. Transfer the pasta to a sizable bowl.
7. Add the kale and pesto. Gently, toss to coat well.

NUTRITION

- Calories: 37
- Fat: 1 g
- Carbs: 3 g
- Fiber: 0 g
- Protein: 4 g
- Sodium: 58 mg

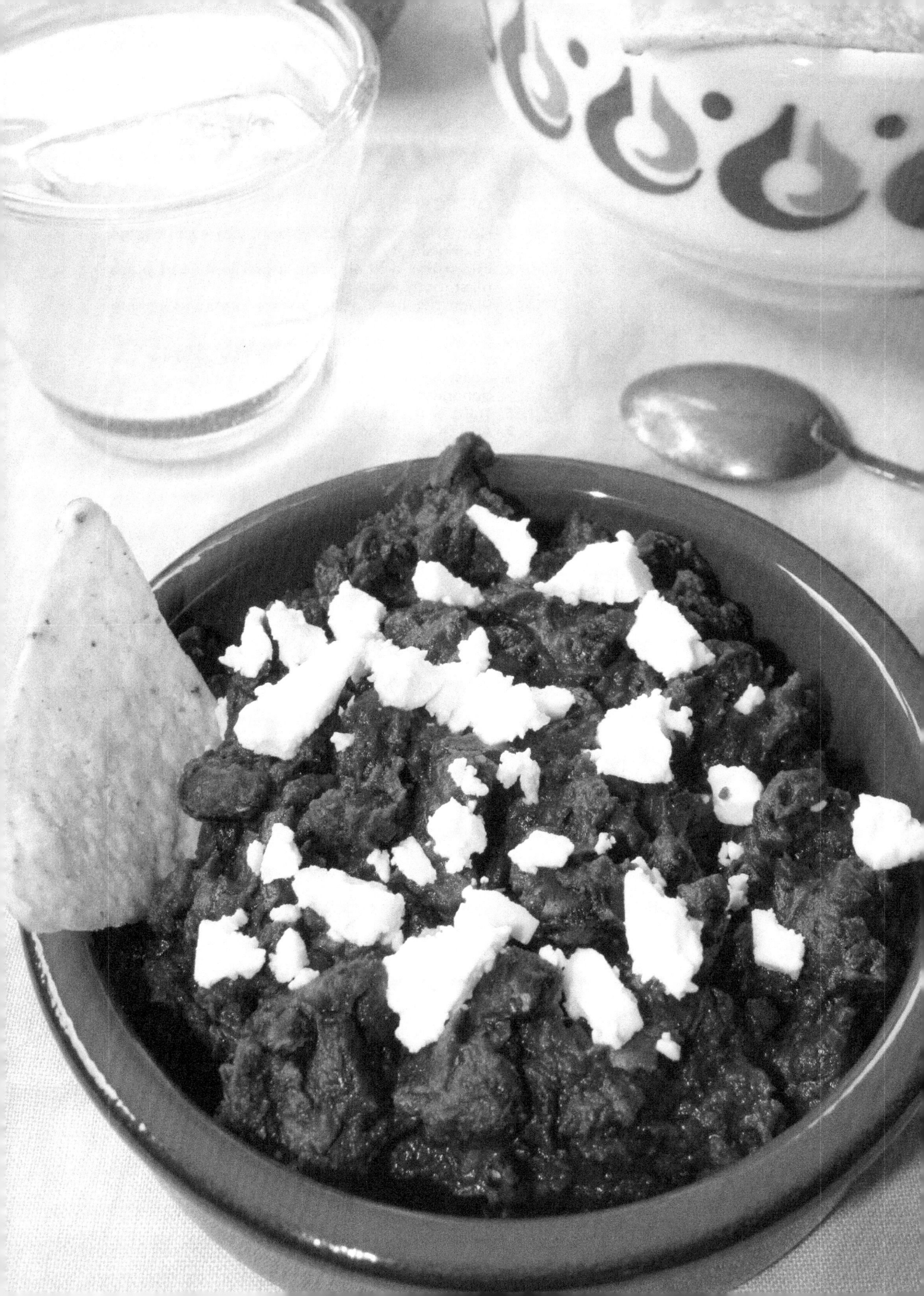

Chapter 9. High-Fiber Recipes

59. Veggie Sandwich

Preparation time: 10 minutes
Cooking time: 0 minutes
Servings: 8

INGREDIENTS

- 2 slices of toasted sprouted-grain bread
- ¼ mashed avocado
- 1 tbsp hummus
- A pinch of salt
- 4 slices cucumber
- 2 slices tomato
- 2 tbsp shredded carrot
- 1 peeled clementine

DIRECTIONS

1. Place one slice of bread onto the plate and spread avocado and hummus.
2. Sprinkle with salt.
3. Fill the sandwich with carrot, tomato, and cucumber.
4. Cut in half and serve with clementine.

NUTRITION

- Calories: 315
- Fat: 10.1 g
- Carbohydrate: 48.6 g
- Protein: 11.4 g
- Fiber: 12.5 g

60. Bean and Veggie Taco Bowl

Preparation time: 20 minutes
Cooking time: 0 minutes
Servings: 1

INGREDIENTS

- 1 tsp olive oil
- ½ cored, and sliced green bell pepper
- ½ sliced red onion
- ½ cup cooked brown rice
- ¼ cup rinsed black beans
- ¼ cup shredded sharp cheddar cheese
- ¼ cup pico de gallo or salsa
- 2 tbsp cilantro

DIRECTIONS

1. Add oil into the skillet and place it over medium flame.
2. Add onion and bell pepper and cook for 5–8 minutes.
3. Mound rice and beans into the bowl. Top with cilantro, pico de gallo, cheese, and vegetables.
4. Top with hot sauce and lime wedges.

NUTRITION

- Calories: 435
- Fat: 15.5 g
- Carbohydrate: 59.6 g
- Protein: 16.4 g
- Fiber: 9.6 g

Preparation time: 10 minutes
Cooking time: 0 minutes
Servings: 1

61. Cobb Salad

INGREDIENTS

- 3 cups chopped iceberg lettuce
- 1 diced, roasted chicken thighs
- 1 stalk, diced celery
- 1 diced carrot
- 1 hard-boiled, diced egg
- 1 tbsp crumbled blue cheese
- 2 tbsp honey and mustard vinaigrette

DIRECTIONS

1. Place blue cheese, egg, carrot, celery, chicken, and lettuce into the salad bowl. Drizzle with dressing

NUTRITION

- Calories: 481
- Fat: 16.7 g
- Carbohydrate: 67.6 g
- Protein: 17.3 g
- Fiber; 13.4 g

Preparation time: 5 minutes
Cooking time: 10 minutes
Servings: 4

62. Asparagus Soup

INGREDIENTS

- 1 tbsp olive oil
- 1 cup chopped shallots
- 3 cloves minced garlic
- 2 lb asparagus, chopped into 1-inch pieces
- 6 cups vegetable stock
- 1 tsp salt

DIRECTIONS

1. Add olive oil into the pot and cook over medium flame. Add garlic and shallot and cook for 3–5 minutes until softened.
2. Add salt, vegetable stock, and asparagus stalks, and then boil it.
3. Cover the pot with a lid and simmer on a low flame.
4. When done, transfer the cooled soup into the blender and blend until creamy.
5. Add asparagus tops and cook for 5 minutes until tender.
6. Serve and enjoy!

NUTRITION

- Calories: 205
- Carbs: 18 g
- Protein: 7 g
- Fat: 0 g
- Fiber: 11 g

Preparation time: 5 minutes
Cooking time: 1 hour
Servings: 6

63. Lentil Soup

INGREDIENTS

- 2 tbsp olive oil
- 1 chopped onion
- 2 chopped carrots
- 2 chopped celery stalks
- 3 potatoes, unpeeled and cubed
- 2 bay leaf
- 2 cups lentils, uncooked and rinsed
- ½ tsp thyme
- ½ tsp oregano
- 5 cups vegetable broth
- 3 cups water

DIRECTIONS

1. Add olive oil into the pot and cook over medium-high flame.
2. Add potatoes, celery, carrots, and onion and cook for 7–8 minutes.
3. Then, add oregano, thyme, lentils, and bay leaves and cook for a few minutes more.
4. Add water and vegetable broth and boil it for 45 minutes until softened.
5. Serve and enjoy!

NUTRITION

- Calories: 229
- Carbs: 30 g
- Protein: 9 g
- Fat: 10 g
- Fiber: 9 g

Preparation time: 5 minutes
Cooking time: 30 minutes
Servings: 4

64. Mushroom Barley Soup

INGREDIENTS

- 2 tbsp olive oil
- 1 cup chopped carrots
- 1 cup chopped onion
- 1 lb sliced white mushrooms
- 1 ½ cup chopped smoked ham
- 28 oz chicken broth
- 14 oz seedless stewed tomatoes
- ½ cup quick-cooking barley

DIRECTIONS

1. Add olive oil into the pot and cook over medium-high flame.
2. Add onion and carrots and cook for 5 minutes.
3. Add mushrooms and cook for 5 minutes more.
4. Add ham and cook for 1–2 minutes and stir well.
5. Add barley, tomatoes, and chicken broth and stir well.
6. Let boil it. Then, lower the heat and simmer for 20 minutes.
7. Serve and enjoy!

NUTRITION

- Calories: 200
- Carbs: 30.8 g
- Protein: 5.8 g
- Fat: 7.3 g
- Fiber: 4.8 g

Preparation time: 5 minutes
Cooking time: 45 minutes
Servings: 4

65. Broccoli Soup

INGREDIENTS

- 2 tbsp olive oil
- 1 chopped leek
- 1 chopped celery stalk
- 2 cloves, minced garlic
- 3 unpeeled, chopped potatoes
- ½ tsp salt
- 1 bay leaf
- 3 cups vegetable broth
- 1 ½ cup broccoli florets

DIRECTIONS

1. Add oil to the pan and cook over medium-high flame.
2. Add bay leaf, salt, potatoes, garlic, leek, and celery, and cook until browned.
3. Add stock and boil it. Then, lower the heat and simmer for 30 minutes.
4. Add broccoli florets and simmer for 15 minutes until tender.
5. Remove from the flame. Let it cool.
6. Discard bay leaf and then add to the blender and blend until smooth.
7. Serve and enjoy!

NUTRITION

- Calories: 361
- Carbs: 33 g
- Protein: 12 g
- Fat: 23 g
- Fiber: 12 g

Preparation time: 5 minutes
Cooking time: 20 minutes
Servings: 4

66. Chicken and Asparagus Pasta

INGREDIENTS

- 1 lb whole-wheat penne pasta
- 2 tbsp olive oil
- 1 lb boneless and sliced into strips chicken breast halves
- ½ tsp poultry seasoning
- 4 cloves, minced garlic
- 1 ½ cup, thawed, cut into 1-inch pieces asparagus, froz en
- 1 cup thawed peas, froz en
- ¼ cup grated Parmesan cheese

DIRECTIONS

1. Add water and salt into the pot and boil it. Then, add pasta and cook until al dente.
2. Add 1 tablespoon of olive oil into the pan and cook over medium flame. Add chicken and poultry seasoning and cook until golden.
3. Remove cooked chicken from the pan.
4. Then, add peas, asparagus, garlic, and the remaining tablespoon of olive oil and cook until tender.
5. Add chicken back with asparagus mixture and cook for 2 minutes.
6. Add pasta to the bowl and toss with chicken mixture.
7. Sprinkle with Parmesan cheese.

NUTRITION

- Calories: 625
- Carbs: 76 g
- Protein: 34 g
- Fat: 23 g
- Fiber: 9 g

Preparation time: 5 minutes
Cooking time: 35 minutes
Servings: 4

67. Red Beans and Rice

INGREDIENTS

- 1 tbsp olive oil
- 1 chopped onion
- 3 chopped celery stalks
- 3 minced garlic cloves
- 14 oz tomato sauce
- ½ tsp oregano
- ½ tbsp thyme
- 14 oz beef stock
- 28 oz drained and rinsed red beans
- 4 cups cooked brown rice

DIRECTIONS

1. Add olive oil into the pan and cook over medium flame.
2. Add garlic, celery, and onions and cook and stir well.
3. Add thyme, oregano, and tomato paste and stir well.
4. Add beef broth and simmer for 35 minutes.
5. Add red beans and cook it well.
6. Place over brown rice.

NUTRITION

- Calories: 413
- Carbs: 76.3 g
- Protein: 21.1 g
- Fat: 2.5 g
- Fiber: 10.1 g

Preparation time: 5 minutes
Cooking time: 35 minutes
Servings: 2-3

68. Beef Stir Fry

INGREDIENTS

- ¼ cup orange juice
- ¼ cup low-sodium soy sauce
- 2 tbsp rice vinegar
- ¼ cup water
- 2 tbsp canola oil
- 8 oz thinly sliced beef round steak
- 3 cloves, minced garlic
- 6 oz peas
- 1 bunch of broccoli florets
- 8 oz shelled edamame
- 1 ½ tsp cornstarch, dissolved in ¼ cup hot water

DIRECTIONS

1. Mix the water, rice vinegar, soy sauce, and orange juice into the bowl and keep it aside.
2. Add 1 tablespoon of canola oil into the pan and cook over medium flame.
3. Add beef and cook for 2 minutes. Transfer the beef to another plate.
4. Add 1 tablespoon of oil into another pan and cook over medium flame.
5. Add garlic and cook for 1 minute. Add edamame, broccoli, and peas, and cook for 3 minutes.
6. Add soy sauce mixture and cook for 5 minutes until tender.
7. Place sliced beef back in the pan.
8. Meanwhile, add cornstarch to the water and dissolve it. Add it to the pan and combine it well.
9. Serve and enjoy!

NUTRITION

- Calories: 368
- Carbs: 27 g
- Protein: 37 g
- Fat: 13 g
- Fiber: 3 g

Preparation time: 10 minutes
Cooking time: 0 minutes
Servings: 2

69. Black Bean Nacho Soup

INGREDIENTS
- 18 oz low-sodium black bean soup
- ¼ tsp smoked paprika
- ½ tsp lime juice
- ½ cup halved grape tomatoes
- ½ cup shredded cabbage
- 2 tbsp cotija cheese
- ½ diced avocado
- 2 oz baked tortilla chips

DIRECTIONS
1. Place soup into the saucepan and then add paprika in it and stir well.
2. Add lime juice and stir and cook it well.
3. Place soup among 2 bowls and top with sliced avocado, cheese, tomatoes, and cabbage.
4. Serve with tortilla chips.

NUTRITION
- Calories: 350
- Carbs: 44.1 g
- Protein: 10.1 g
- Fat: 16.9 g
- Fiber: 9.4 g

Preparation time: 15 minutes
Cooking time: 0 minutes
Servings: 1

70. Butternut Squash Soup

INGREDIENTS
- 15 oz butternut squash soup
- ¾ cup rinsed chickpeas
- 1 tbsp lime juice
- 1 tsp curry powder
- A pinch of salt
- 2 tbsp diced avocado
- 1 tbsp non-fat plain Greek yogurt

DIRECTIONS
1. Add soup into the saucepan and heat it.
2. Add salt, curry powder, lime juice, and chickpeas and stir and cook it.
3. When done, top with yogurt and avocado.

NUTRITION
- Calories: 402
- Carbs: 67.7 g
- Protein: 16.1 g
- Fat: 8.8 g
- Fiber: 13.4 g

Preparation time: 20 minutes
Cooking time: 0 minutes
Servings: 5

71. Broccoli Salad

INGREDIENTS

- ½ cup mayonnaise
- 1 tbsp whole-grain mustard
- 1 tbsp cider vinegar
- 1 grated garlic clove
- 1 tsp sugar
- ¼ tsp ground pepper
- 4 cups chopped broccoli crowns
- 1 cup chopped cauliflower
- ¼ cup chopped red onion
- 3 tbsp toasted sunflower seeds

DIRECTIONS

1. Add pepper, sugar, garlic, vinegar, mustard, and mayonnaise into the bowl and whisk it well.
2. Add sunflower seeds, onion, broccoli, and cauliflower and stir well.
3. Serve and enjoy!

NUTRITION

- Calories: 246
- Carbs: 7.7 g
- Protein: 5.4 g
- Fat: 2.8 g
- Fiber: 22 g

Preparation time: 20 minutes
Cooking time: 0 minutes
Servings: 4

72. Beef and Bean Sloppy Joes

INGREDIENTS

- 1 tbsp extra-virgin olive oil
- 12 oz ground beef
- 1 cup rinsed no-salt-added black beans
- 1 cup chopped onion
- 2 tsp chili powder
- ½ tsp garlic powder
- ½ tsp onion powder
- Pinch of cayenne pepper
- 1 cup tomato sauce
- 3 tbsp ketchup
- 1 tbsp Worcestershire sauce
- 2 tsp spicy brown mustard
- 1 tsp brown sugar
- 4 split and toasted whole-wheat hamburger buns

DIRECTIONS

1. Add oil into the skillet and cook over medium-high flame.
2. Add beef and cook for 3–4 minutes until browned.
3. Transfer the beef to the bowl using a slotted spoon.
4. Add onion and beans to the pan and cook until softened for 5 minutes.
5. Add cayenne, onion powder, garlic powder, and chili powder, and cook for 30 seconds.
6. Add brown sugar, mustard, Worcestershire sauce, ketchup, and tomato sauce, and stir well. Place beef back in the pan and simmer for 5 minutes.
7. Serve and enjoy!

NUTRITION

- Calories: 411
- Carbs: 43.8 g
- Protein: 25.8 g
- Fat: 15 g
- Fiber: 8.4 g

Preparation time: 15 minutes
Baking time: 20 minutes
Servings: 6

73. Sweet Potato and Peanut Soup

INGREDIENTS

- 2 tbsp canola oil
- 1 ½ cup diced yellow onion
- 1 tbsp minced garlic
- 1 tbsp minced fresh ginger
- 4 tsp red curry paste
- 1 minced Serrano chili, ribs and seeds removed
- 1 lb peeled and cubed sweet potatoes
- 3 cups water
- 1 cup coconut milk
- ¾ cup unsalted dry-roasted peanuts
- 15 oz rinsed white beans
- ¾ tsp salt
- ¼ tsp ground pepper
- ¼ cup chopped fresh cilantro
- 2 tbsp lime juice
- ¼ cup unsalted roasted pumpkin seeds
- Lime wedges to garnish

DIRECTIONS

1. Add oil into the pot and heat over medium-high flame.
2. Add onion and cook until softened.
3. Add Serrano, curry paste, ginger, and garlic and stir and cook for 1 minute. Add water and sweet potatoes and boil them.
4. Lower the heat and cook over medium-low flame for 10–12 minutes.
5. Transfer half of the soup to the blender and then add peanut and coconut milk and blend until smooth. Place it back in the pot with the remaining soup.
6. Add pepper, salt, and beans and stir well.
7. When done, remove from the flame.
8. Add lime juice and fresh cilantro leaves.
9. Serve and enjoy!

NUTRITION

- Calories: 345
- Carbs: 37.4 g
- Protein: 12.6 g
- Fat: 19.4 g
- Fiber: 8.4 g

Preparation time: 15 minutes
Baking time: 1 hour and 10 minutes
Servings: 6

74. Beet Salad

INGREDIENTS

- 2 lb scrubbed beets
- 3 tbsp extra-virgin olive oil
- 2 tbsp balsamic vinegar
- ¼ tsp salt
- ¼ tsp ground pepper
- ⅓ cup crumbled Feta cheese
- 2 tbsp chopped fresh dill

DIRECTIONS

1. Preheat the oven to 400°F.
2. Wrap beets in the foil and put them onto the rimmed baking sheet.
3. Bake for 1 hour and 10 minutes until tender.
4. Let it cool. Peel and cut into cubes.
5. Whisk the pepper, salt, vinegar, and oil into the bowl.
6. Add Feta and beets and toss to combine.
7. Top with dill.

NUTRITION

- Calories: 155
- Carbs: 15.8 g
- Protein: 3.7 g
- Fat: 9 g
- Fiber: 4.3 g

Preparation time: 10 minutes
Cooking time: 1 hour and 5 minutes
Servings: 6

75. Broccoli Casserole

INGREDIENTS

- 2 slices of whole-wheat sandwich bread
- 2 lb broccoli florets
- 3 tbsp butter
- 2 tbsp extra-virgin olive oil
- 2 cups diced onion
- 4 cloves minced garlic
- ⅓ cup all-purpose flour
- 3 ½ cups low-sodium chicken broth
- 6 oz low-fat cream cheese
- 2 tsp Worcestershire sauce
- ¾ tsp ground pepper
- ½ tsp salt
- 2 cups shredded Colby Jack cheese

NUTRITION

- Calories: 225
- Carbs: 13.1 g
- Protein: 10.9 g
- Fat: 15.1 g
- Fiber: 3.2 g

DIRECTIONS

1. Preheat the oven to 300°F.
2. Let coat the baking dish with cooking spray.
3. Add bread into pieces and then add to the food processor until crumbs form.
4. Place breadcrumbs onto the baking sheet and bake for 10 minutes.
5. During this, add water to the pot and boil it. Add broccoli and steam it for 4–6 minutes. Let chop it and place it onto the baking dish.
6. Elevate the temperature to 350°F.
7. Add oil and 1 tablespoon of butter into the saucepan and cook over medium-high flame. Add garlic and onion and cook for 3–5 minutes.
8. Place flour over the vegetables and cook for 1 minute.
9. Add chicken broth and stir well. Let cook for 3 minutes.
10. Add salt, pepper, Worcestershire sauce, and cream cheese and stir well. Cook for 2 minutes.
11. Remove from the flame. Add cheese and stir well.
12. Place cheese sauce onto the broccoli.
13. Melt 2 tbsp of butter and mix with breadcrumbs into the bowl.
14. Place over the broccoli mixture and top with a half cup of cheese.
15. Bake for 25–30 minutes.
16. Serve and enjoy!

Dinner recipes

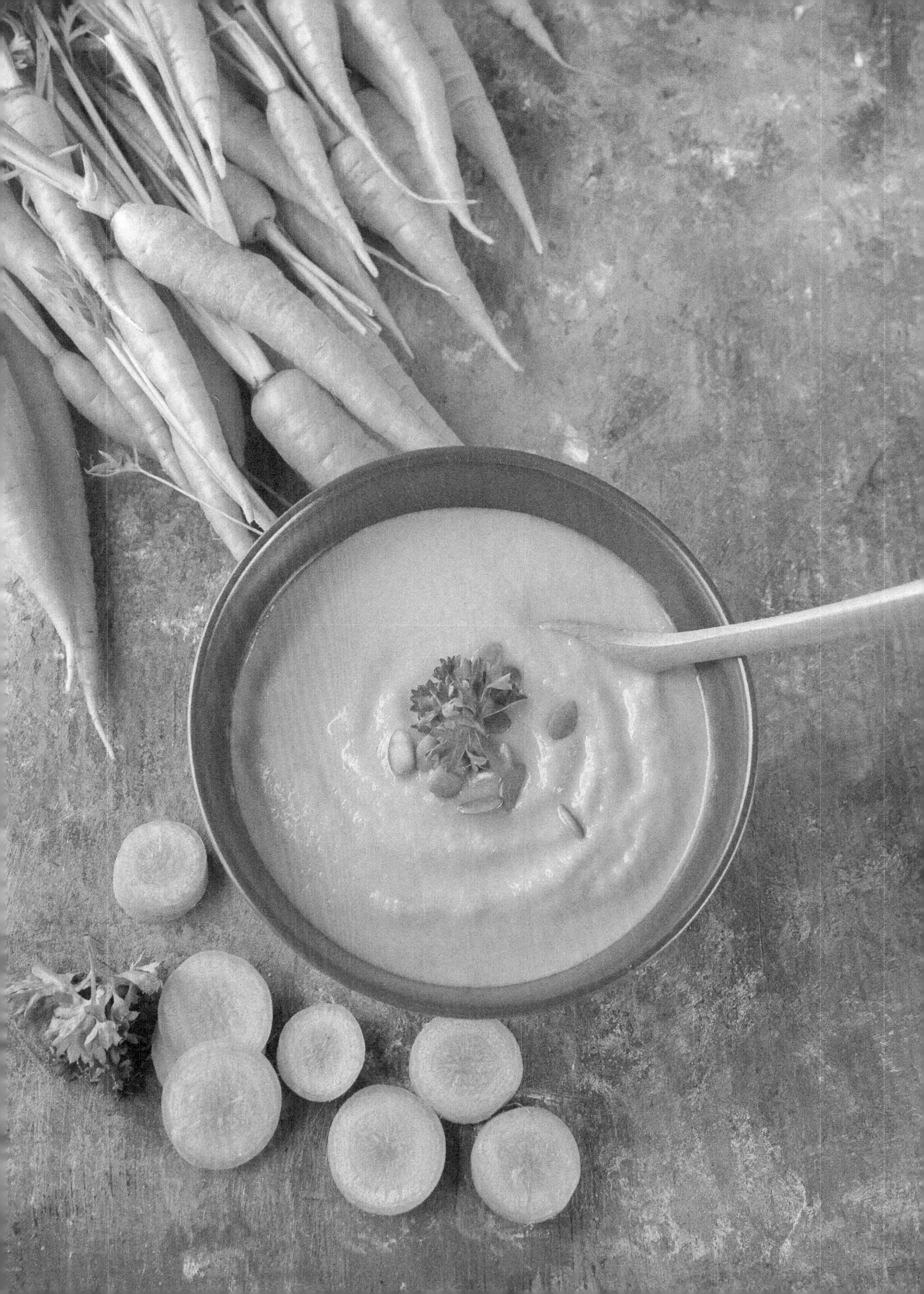

Chapter 10. Clear Liquid Recipes

Preparation time: 20 minutes
Cooking time: 40 minutes
Servings: 4

76. Beet Soup

INGREDIENTS
- 3 tbsp olive oil
- 1 chopped onion
- 3 chopped garlic cloves
- 6 peeled and chopped beets
- 2 cups beef stock
- Salt and freshly ground pepper to taste
- Heavy cream

DIRECTIONS
1. Add olive oil into the saucepan and heat it over medium flame.
2. Then, add garlic and onion and stir well. Let cook for 5 minutes until soft. Add beets and cook for 1 minute.
3. Add pepper, salt, and stock, and stir well. Let boil it for 20–30 minutes. Remove from the flame. Let it cool.
4. Add soup into the food processor and blend until smooth.
5. Place soup back in the saucepan and heat it.
6. Then, place it into the bowls. Garnish with sour cream.

NUTRITION
- Calories: 229
- Carbs: 17 g
- Protein: 4.8 g
- Fat: 16.4 g

Preparation time: 10 minutes
Cooking time: 10 minutes
Servings: 4

77. Chicken Burgers

INGREDIENTS
- 1 lb extra-lean ground chicken
- ½ cup bread crumbs
- ½ grated onion
- 1 egg
- 2 cloves, minced garlic
- Salt and ground black pepper to taste
- 2 tsp olive oil

DIRECTIONS
1. Combine the black pepper, salt, garlic, egg, onion, ground chicken, and ¼ cup of breadcrumbs into the bowl.
2. Make patties from the mixture.
3. Place the remaining ¼ cup of breadcrumbs into the dish and roll the patties into the breadcrumbs.
4. Add olive oil into the skillet and cook over medium-high flame.
5. Place patties in the oil and cook for 5–6 minutes.
6. Turnover and cook for 3–4 minutes.
7. Serve and enjoy!

NUTRITION
- Calories: 238
- Carbs: 11.5 g
- Protein: 28.8 g
- Fat: 7.8 g

Preparation time: 15 minutes
Cooking time: 25 minutes
Servings: 4

78. Fresh Asparagus Soup

INGREDIENTS

- 1 lb fresh asparagus, trimmed and cut into 1-inch pieces
- ½ cup chopped onion
- 14.5-oz chicken broth
- 2 tbsp butter
- 2 tbsp all-purpose flour
- 1 tsp salt
- A pinch of ground black pepper
- 1 cup milk
- ½ cup sour cream
- 1 tsp fresh lemon juice

DIRECTIONS

1. Add half a cup of chicken broth, chopped onion, and asparagus into the saucepan and cook over high flame. Lower the heat and cook for 12 minutes more until tender.
2. Add mixture into the blender and blend until smooth. Keep it aside.
3. Add butter into the saucepan and cook over medium-low flame.
4. Add pepper, salt, and flour and stir and cook for 2 minutes.
5. Add the remaining chicken broth and whisk it well. Elevate the heat to medium and cook and stir well. Then, add milk and asparagus puree to it.
6. Add sour cream into the bowl. Then, add a ladleful of the hot soup to the sour cream and stir well. Place lemon juice and sour cream mixture into the soup and mix well.
7. Serve and enjoy!

NUTRITION

- Calories: 196
- Carbs: 14.1 g
- Protein: 6.6 g
- Fat: 13.4 g

Preparation time: 10 minutes
Cooking time: 20 minutes
Servings: 12

79. Pumpkin Waffles

INGREDIENTS

Dry ingredients:

- 2 cups all-purpose flour
- ¼ cup brown sugar
- 1 tsp baking powder
- ½ tsp baking soda
- ¼ tsp salt
- 1–2 tsp pumpkin spice
- 1 tsp cinnamon

Wet ingredients:

- 3 eggs
- 1 ⅓ cup milk
- ¼ cup maple syrup
- 3 tbsp oil or melted butter
- 1 cup pumpkin

DIRECTIONS

1. Add dry ingredients into the bowl and stir well.
2. Whisk the melted butter, pumpkin, maple syrup, milk, and eggs into the jug
3. Add wet ingredients to the dry ingredients and combine them well.
4. Place mixture into the waffle maker and bake for 20 minutes.
5. When done, serve and enjoy!

NUTRITION

- Calories: 183
- Carbs: 28 g
- Protein: 5 g
- Fat: 6 g

Preparation time: 5 minutes
Cooking time: 1 hour 15 minutes
Servings: 8

80. Bean Soup

INGREDIENTS
- 16 oz beans
- 7 cups water
- 1 ham bone
- 2 cups diced ham
- ¼ cup minced onion
- ½ tsp salt
- A pinch of ground black pepper
- 1 bay leaf
- ½ cup sliced carrots
- ½ cup sliced celery

DIRECTIONS
1. Add rinsed beans into the pot and then add water and boil it for 2 minutes.
2. When done, remove from the flame. Cover with a lid and let sit for 1 hour.
3. Add bay leaves, pepper, salt, onion, cubed ham, and ham bone and boil it. Lower the heat and simmer for 1 hour and 15 minutes.
4. Add celery and carrots and cook until tender.
5. Remove bone and ham bone and place them back in the soup.
6. Serve and enjoy!

NUTRITION
- Calories: 247
- Carbs: 36.7 g
- Protein: 17.4 g
- Fat: 3.8 g

Preparation time: 20 minutes
Cooking time: 0 minutes
Chill time: 4 hours
Servings: 4

81. Carrot Cucumber Salad

INGREDIENTS
- ¼ cup rice wine vinegar
- 2 tbsp snipped fresh cilantro
- 1 tbsp toasted sesame oil
- ¼ tsp salt
- ⅛ tsp chili powder
- ⅛ tsp black pepper
- 1 cucumber, halved lengthwise and cut into slices
- 2 carrots, cut into matchstick-size pieces
- ½ red onion, thinly sliced

DIRECTIONS
1. Add black pepper, chili powder, salt, oil, cilantro, and vinegar into the bowl and whisk it well.
2. Add red onion, carrots, and cucumber and stir well. Toss to combine.
3. Let it chill for 2–4 hours.
4. Serve!

NUTRITION
- Calories: 60
- Carbs: 8.2 g
- Protein: 0.9 g
- Fat: 3.6 g

Preparation time: 5 minutes
Cooking time: 20 minutes
Servings: 4

82. Lemon Chicken and Rice

INGREDIENTS

- 2 tbsp butter
- 1 lb chicken breasts, cut into strips, boneless and skinless
- 1 chopped onion
- 1 thinly sliced carrot
- 2 minced garlic cloves
- 1 tbsp cornstarch
- 14 oz chicken broth
- 2 tbsp lemon juice
- ¼ tsp salt
- 1 cup froz en peas
- 1 ½ cup uncooked instant rice

DIRECTIONS

1. Add butter into the skillet and cook over medium-high flame.
2. Then, add garlic, carrot, chicken, and onion and cook for 5–7 minutes.
3. Combine the salt, lemon juice, broth, and cornstarch into the bowl, and then add to the skillet. Let cook and stir for 1–2 minutes.
4. Add peas and rice and stir well.
5. When done, remove from the flame.
6. Let stand for 5 minutes.
7. Serve and enjoy!

NUTRITION

- Calories: 370
- Carbs: 41 g
- Protein: 29 g
- Fat: 9 g

Preparation time: 5 minutes
Cooking time: 20 minutes
Servings: 4

83. Peachy Pork with Rice

INGREDIENTS

- 1 cup cooked brown rice
- 1 lb cut into 1-inch cubes pork tenderloin
- 2 tbsp olive oil
- 2 tbsp low-sodium taco seasoning
- 1 cup salsa
- 3 tbsp peach preserves

DIRECTIONS

1. Add pork into the bowl and drizzle with oil. Sprinkle with taco seasoning and toss to combine.
2. Add pork into the skillet and cook for 8–10 minutes.
3. Add peach preserve and salsa and stir well.
4. Serve with cooked rice.

NUTRITION

- Calories: 387
- Carbs: 42 g
- Protein: 25 g
- Fat: 12 g

Preparation time: 10 minutes
Cooking time: 25 minutes
Servings: 2

84. Loaded Pumpkin Chowder

INGREDIENTS

- 200 g pumpkin puree, mashed, peeled, and boiled
- 200 ml water
- 200 g pumpkin, peeled, boiled, and cut into chunks
- 1 peeled and julienned carrot
- 2 tbsp extra-virgin olive oil
- 1 pre-cooked chicken breast
- ½ cup chopped baby spinach
- 1 tsp celery powder
- 1 low-salted chicken stock cube
- 1 bay leaf
- Salt and pepper to taste

DIRECTIONS

1. Add olive oil into the saucepan and heat it.
2. Add water, bay leaf, celery powder, and pureed pumpkin and simmer for 10 minutes.
3. Add pumpkin chunks and shredded chicken to the pan and bring to simmer for 5–7 minutes.
4. Add baby spinach and julienned carrot and cook for 5 minutes.
5. Discard bay leaf.
6. Serve!

NUTRITION

- Calories: 127
- Carbs: 22 g
- Fat: 2 g
- Protein: 5 g
- Fiber: 4 g

Preparation time: 10 minutes
Cooking time: 30 minutes
Servings: 4

85. Creamy Carrot Soup

INGREDIENTS

- 1 tbsp olive oil or butter
- 4 slices of streaky bacon
- 1 chopped onion
- 2 minced garlic cloves
- 5 cut into chunks carrots
- 4 cups vegetable or chicken broth
- ¼ cup creams
- ¾ cup milk
- Salt and pepper to taste

For the servings:

- Chopped fresh thyme or parsley

For the swirling cream:

- Crusty bread

DIRECTIONS

1. Add oil into the pot and cook over medium-high flame.
2. Add bacon and cook until golden. Remove from the pot. Let it cool.
3. Add garlic and onion to the bacon dripping and cook for 2 minutes.
4. Add carrots and stir well.
5. Then, add broth and stir well. Cover with a lid and cook for 20–25 minutes.
6. Remove the lid from the flame.
7. Add carrot into the blender and blend until smooth.
8. Add pepper, salt, milk, and cream and stir well.
9. Place soup into the bowls.
10. Garnish with fresh parsley or thyme.

NUTRITION

- Calories: 351
- Carbs: 16 g
- Protein: 11 g
- Fat: 27 g

Preparation time: 10 minutes
Cooking time: 20 minutes
Servings: 4

86. Fish Stew

INGREDIENTS

- 6 tbsp extra-virgin olive oil
- 1 chopped onion
- 3 minced garlic cloves
- ⅔ cup chopped fresh parsley leaves
- 1 ½ cup chopped tomato
- 2 tsp optional tomato paste
- 1 cup clam juice
- ½ cup dry white wine
- 1 ½ lb fish fillets, cut into pieces
- A pinch of dried oregano
- A pinch of dried thyme
- ⅛ tsp Tabasco sauce
- ⅛ tsp freshly ground black pepper
- 1 tsp salt

DIRECTIONS

1. Add olive oil into the pot and cook over medium-high flame.
2. Add onion and cook for 4 minutes. Then, add garlic and cook for 1 minute more. Then, add parsley and cook for 2 minutes more.
3. Add tomato paste and tomato and cook for 10 minutes more.
4. Add fish, dry white wine, and clam juice and simmer for 3–5 minutes. Then, place Tabasco, thyme, oregano, pepper, and salt.
5. Sprinkle with pepper and salt if needed. Place soup into the bowls.
6. Serve and enjoy!

NUTRITION

- Calories: 389
- Carbs: 7 g
- Protein: 33 g
- Fat: 23 g

Preparation time: 10 minutes
Cooking time: 30 minutes
Servings: 4

87. Mushroom Soup

INGREDIENTS

- 4 tbsp butter
- 1 tbsp oil
- 2 diced onions
- 4 cloves minced garlic
- 1 ½ lb mushrooms, sliced fresh brown
- 4 tsp chopped thyme
- ½ cup white wine
- 6 tbsp all-purpose flour
- 4 cups low-sodium chicken broth or stock
- 1–2 tsp salt
- ½–1 tsp black cracked pepper
- 2 crumbled beef bouillon cubes
- 1 cup heavy cream
- Fresh parsley and thyme to serve, chopped

DIRECTIONS

1. Add oil and butter into the pot and cook over medium-high flame.
2. Then, add onion and cook for 2–3 minutes. Add garlic and cook for 1 minute more.
3. Add 2 tsp thyme and mushrooms and cook for 5 minutes.
4. Add wine and cook for 3 minutes.
5. Add flour over the mushrooms and cook for 2 minutes. Add stock and combine it well. Lower the heat and sprinkle with bouillon cubes, pepper, and salt.
6. Let simmer for 10–15 minutes.
7. Lower the heat and then add cream and stir well.
8. Sprinkle with pepper and salt if needed.
9. Sprinkle with fresh parsley and thyme.

NUTRITION

- Calories: 271
- Carbs: 21 g
- Protein: 8 g
- Fat: 13 g

Preparation time: 10 minutes
Cooking time: 30 minutes
Servings: 10

88. Chicken Soup

INGREDIENTS
- 3 lb whole chicken
- 4 halved carrots
- 4 celery stalks, halved
- 1 halved onion
- Water to cover
- Salt and pepper to taste
- 1 tsp chicken bouillon granules

DIRECTIONS
1. Add onion, celery, carrots, and chicken into the pot and then add cold water and simmer until chicken is tender.
2. Remove all content from the pot and then strain it through a strainer.
3. Chop the onion, celery, and carrots and remove the bones from the meat. Sprinkle with chicken bouillon, pepper, and salt.
4. Place onion, chicken, carrots, and celery back in the pot.
5. Stir and serve!

NUTRITION
- Calories: 152
- Fat: 8.9 g
- Carbs: 4.2 g
- Protein: 13.1 g

Preparation time: 5 minutes
Cooking time: 1 hour
Servings: 11

89. Pumpkin Casserole

INGREDIENTS
- 2 cups pumpkin puree
- 1 cup evaporated milk
- 1 cup white sugar
- ½ cup self-rising flour
- 2 eggs
- 1 tsp vanilla extract
- ½ cup butter
- 2 pinches of ground cinnamon

DIRECTIONS
1. Preheat the oven to 350°F.
2. Mix the ground cinnamon, melted butter, vanilla, eggs, flour, sugar, pumpkin, and evaporated milk. Place mixture into the casserole dish.
3. Place it into the oven and bake for one hour.
4. Serve and enjoy!

NUTRITION
- Calories: 219
- Fat: 11 g
- Carbs: 27.2 g
- Protein: 3.7 g

90. Fresh Tomato Juice

Preparation time: 15 minutes
Cooking time: 40 minutes
Servings: 12

INGREDIENTS

- 10 lb washed, quartered, and cores removed tomatoes
- Salt and black pepper to taste
- 6 ½ tbsp lemon juice
- Pepper, onion powder, paprika, cayenne, celery salt, chili powder, or hot sauce (optional)

DIRECTIONS

1. Prepare all ingredients.
2. Add tomatoes into the saucepan and simmer for 30 minutes until tender.
3. Place strainer over the bowl. Add tomatoes and separate the juice, seeds, skins, and chunks.
4. Place the remaining juice back in the pan and heat it.
5. Add pepper, lemon juice, and salt and boil it. Add optional seasoning if you want.
6. When done, transfer juice to the glass.

NUTRITION

- Calories: 69
- Carbs: 15 g
- Protein: 3 g
- Fat: 1 g

---

91. Ground Beef Tostada

Preparation time: 15 minutes
Cooking time: 50 minutes
Servings: 8

INGREDIENTS

- 1 ½ lb ground beef
- 1 tsp salt
- 1 tbsp chili powder
- 1 tsp oregano
- 1 tsp ground cumin
- 1 diced white onion
- 2 seeded and diced jalapeños
- ¼ cup tomato paste
- 16 oz roasted tomatoes, diced
- 2 peeled and diced carrots
- 1 diced Yukon gold potato

For the assemble:
- Tostadas
- 2 cups refried beans
- Cotija cheese
- Sour cream
- Pickled red onions
- Cilantro chopped

DIRECTIONS

1. Add cumin, chili powder, oregano, salt, kosher salt, and ground beef into the stockpot and cook over medium-high flame. Let cook for 6–7 minutes.
2. Then, add tomato paste, jalapenos, and onion and stir well. Cook for a few minutes more. Then, add tomatoes and their juices and lower the heat and cook for 20 minutes.
3. Add carrot and diced potatoes and cook for 20 minutes more. Stir well. Add water if it gets too thick.
4. Assemble: Place refried beans onto the tostada and top with ground beef mixture. Then, add chopped cilantro, pickled red onion, and sour cream.

NUTRITION

- Calories: 235
- Carbs: 10 g
- Protein: 19 g
- Fat: 12 g

92. Beef Barley Soup

Preparation time: 10 minutes
Cooking time: 1 hour 10 minutes
Servings: 6

INGREDIENTS

- 2 tsp olive oil
- 1 lb ground beef
- 1 cup chopped onion
- ½ tbsp minced garlic
- 3 peeled and sliced carrots
- ½ cup dry barley
- 2-3 bay leaves
- 2 cups tomato sauce
- 1 tbsp soy sauce
- 1 tbsp miso paste
- 2 cups water
- 1 tbsp fresh parsley for garnish

DIRECTIONS

1. Add olive oil into the pot and cook over medium-high flame for 2 minutes. Add ground beef and cook for 5-7 minutes until browned.
2. Then, add garlic and onion and cook for 3-4 minutes more.
3. Add bay leaves, barley, carrots, and stir well, and cook for 2 minutes.
4. Add water, miso paste, soy sauce, and tomato sauce and stir well.
5. Let simmer for 1 hour.
6. Garnish with fresh parsley leaves.

NUTRITION

- Calories: 234
- Carbs: 28.6 g
- Protein: 21.2 g
- Fat: 4.7 g

93. Ground Beef and Rice Bowls

Preparation time: 5 minutes
Cooking time: 15 minutes
Servings: 4

INGREDIENTS

- 1 lb lean ground beef
- 3 minced garlic cloves
- ¼ cup brown sugar
- ¼ cup low-sodium soy sauce
- 2 tsp sesame oil
- ¼ tsp ground ginger
- ¼ tsp crushed red pepper flakes
- ¼ tsp pepper
- 2 cups hot cooked white or brown rice
- Sliced green onions and sesame seeds for garnish

DIRECTIONS

1. Add ground beef into the skillet and cook over medium flame until no longer pink.
2. Whisk the pepper, red pepper flakes, sesame oil, soy sauce, and brown sugar into the bowl.
3. Place this mixture over the ground beef and simmer for 1-2 minutes.
4. Garnish with sesame seeds and green onions.

NUTRITION

- Calories: 238
- Carbs: 16 g
- Protein: 25 g
- Fat: 8 g

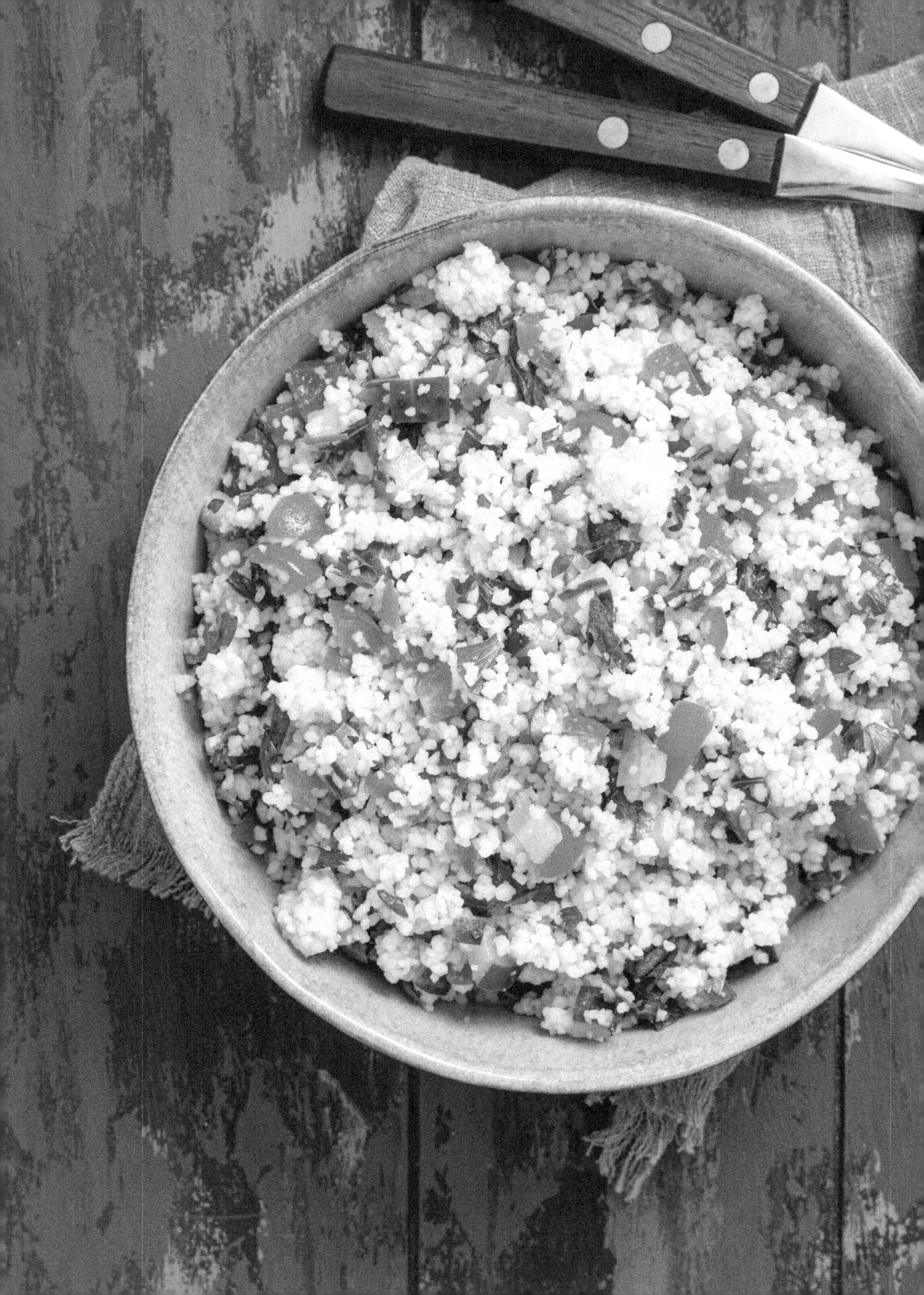

Chapter 11. Low-Residue Recipes

Preparation time: 3 minutes
Cooking time: 4 minutes
Servings: 4

94. Grilled Vegetable Quesadilla

INGREDIENTS

- 1 Zucchini, sliced in half, lengthwise
- 1 Yellow squash, sliced in half lengthwise
- 1 Onion, sliced in fourths, lengthwise
- 1 Red pepper, seeded and quartered
- 2 Portobello mushroom cap
- ½ tsp Italian seasoning
- ¼ tsp salt
- 4 Whole wheat tortillas
- ½ cup Mozzarella cheese, shredded

DIRECTIONS

1. Fry the veggies over moderate flame until they are fully done. Season to taste with salt and Italian spice. Mix the veggies after slicing them.
2. Throw one taco in a pan coated with cooking spray over moderate flame. Cover with part of the veggie combination, cheese, and the other tortilla. Warm the opposite side of the tortillas till the melty cheese, but just don't brown it. Serve.

NUTRITION

- Calories: 227
- Protein 16.8 g
- Carbs 35.6 g
- Fat 14 g

Preparation time: 5 minutes
Cooking time: 4 minutes
Servings: 4

95. Grilled Veggie Sandwich

INGREDIENTS

- 2 Eggplant, sliced into ½-inch-thick slices
- 1 Zucchini, sliced into ½-inch-thick slices
- 1 Red pepper, seeded and quartered
- 2 Portobello mushroom caps
- ½ cup olive oil
- ¼ tsp salt
- 1 cup goat cheese
- 8 oz whole-wheat crusty bread like baguette
- 1 cup fresh baby spinach washed and dried.

DIRECTIONS

1. Coat the veggie pieces and the mushroom tops in olive oil using a pastry cutter. Using salt, flavor them.
2. Sauté until the veggies are soft on a hot grill. Cut the mushroom into ¼-inch pieces, sprinkle goat cheese on both sides of the toast, and cover with 1 piece each of toasted veggies and a fourth of the mushroom to construct.
3. Place the remaining slice of bread on top of the spinach. Serve.

NUTRITION

- Calories: 560
- Protein: 8.3 g
- Carbs: 45 g
- Fat: 40 g

Preparation time: 5 minutes
Cooking time: 4 minutes
Servings: 4

96. Lentil Linguine Stew

INGREDIENTS

- 3 tsp olive oil
- 1 Onion, chopped
- 1 tbsp Garlic cloves, minced
- 1 Carrots, chopped
- 2 Celery stalks, chopped
- 1 cup lentils, uncooked, rinsed
- 6 cups vegetable broth
- 4 cups water
- 2 tsp salt
- 3 Bay leaves
- ½ cup linguine, cut into 1-inch pieces
- 2 cups kale, chopped
- ½ cup Italian parsley, chopped

DIRECTIONS

1. Warm the canola oil in a big saucepan over low heat. Cook for 10 minutes, tossing periodically, until the onion, garlic, carrots, and celery are soft.
2. Combine the lentils, broth, water, salt, and bay leaf in a large mixing bowl. Raise the temperature to be high and bring the mixture to a boil. Reduce the heat to low and cook for 25 minutes, slightly covered.
3. Cook, stirring periodically, for another 15-20 minutes, or until lentils are soft and the pasta and greens are tender.
4. In a large mixing bowl, combine the parsley, salt, and pepper. Serve.

NUTRITION

- Calories: 284
- Protein: 11.6 g
- Carbs: 55 g
- Fat: 1.4 g

Preparation time: 5 minutes
Cooking time: 4 minutes
Servings: 4

97. Lentil Risotto

INGREDIENTS

- 2 tsp olive oil
- Medium leeks, chopped
- Garlic cloves, minced
- Red bell pepper, seeded and chopped
- 3 cups chicken broth
- 1 ¼ cup long grain rice
- 1 tsp fresh basil, chopped
- 1 cup lentils, cooked
- ¼ cup Italian parsley, chopped
- ¼ cup Parmesan cheese, grated

DIRECTIONS

1. Sauté leeks, garlic, and red pepper in olive oil till soft in a medium skillet on medium heat.
2. Combine the broth, rice, and basil in a large mixing bowl. Covered and boil till rice is done, then tossed in prepared lentils for 10 minutes.
3. Take the pan off the heat and stir in the parsley and Parmesan cheese. Serve.

NUTRITION

- Calories: 334
- Protein: 12 g
- Carbs: 41 g
- Fat: 14 g

Preparation time: 4 minutes
Cooking time: 6 minutes
Servings: 4

98. Lentil Stew

INGREDIENTS

- 1 tsp vegetable oil,
- 1 onion, chopped
- 2 garlic cloves, minced
- 1 green bell pepper, chopped
- 2 cups kale, chopped
- 3 cups vegetable broth
- 1 ¼ cup lentils, uncooked, rinsed
- 15 oz can of tomato sauce
- 1 tsp Italian seasoning
- ½ tsp paprika

DIRECTIONS

1. Oil in a large frying small saucepan. Sauté, turning regularly, until onions, garlic, and bell pepper are soft.
2. Put the water, lentils, pasta sauce, and seasonings in a bowl and mix. Lower to a lower thermal setting and partly cover for 35–40 minutes, or till lentils are cooked. Serve.

NUTRITION

- Calories: 120
- Protein: 8.1 g
- Carbs: 22 g
- Fat: 0.5 g

Preparation time: 5 minutes
Cooking time: 4 minutes
Servings: 4

99. Pasta with Beans and Turkey

INGREDIENTS

- 1 lb whole-wheat pasta
- 1 tsp olive oil
- 1 Onion
- 1 tbsp. Garlic cloves, minced
- 1 lb ground turkey
- 1 Small head escarole, rinsed, drained, and chopped
- 14 oz can of cannellini beans, drained and rinsed
- 1 ½ cup chicken broth
- 1 tsp fresh rosemary, chopped
- ½ tsp salt
- ½ tsp pepper
- ½ cup Parmesan cheese

DIRECTIONS

1. A huge kettle of salted water is brought to a boil. Cook pasta as directed on the packet. Drain.
2. On medium-high heat, warm the olive oil in a big pan. Simmer till the onions have softened, then add garlic, and turkey and stir for another 5–7 minutes, or until the turkey has browned.
3. Simmer for 5 minutes, or until the escarole has wilted. 1 cup chicken stock, rosemary, season, and pepper are added to the beans. Cook, occasionally stirring, until the sauce has thickened somewhat.
4. Combine the spaghetti with the turkey-bean combination, adding more chicken stock if required to thin the sauce.
5. Parmigiano cheese should be sprinkled on top. Serve.

NUTRITION

- Calories: 235.6
- Protein: 14.1 g
- Carbs: 36 g
- Fat: 2.6 g

Preparation time: 10 minutes
Cooking time: 5 minutes
Servings: 4

100. Pasta with Spinach and White Beans

INGREDIENTS

- 1 lb whole-wheat pasta
- 2 tsp olive oil
- 1 tbsp. Garlic cloves, minced
- 3 cups tomatoes, chopped
- 14 oz can of cannellini beans, drained and rinsed
- 1 cup tomato sauce
- 2 cups fresh spinach, chopped
- ½ cup Feta cheese, crumbled

DIRECTIONS

1. A big pot of water should be brought to a boil. Season with salt, then add the pasta and cook according to package directions. Drain.
2. Heat the olive oil in a big pan over medium heat. Cook for 3-4 minutes, depending on the size of the garlic cloves. Combine the tomatoes, beans, and tomato sauce in a large mixing bowl. Bring the water to a boil. Reduce heat to low, cover, and cook for 20 minutes.
3. Allow the sauce to boil for another 5 minutes, or until the spinach has wilted. Spread sauce over hot pasta in a generous portion dish and top with Feta cheese. Toss everything together. Serve.

NUTRITION

- Calories: 332
- Protein: 15.8 g
- Carbs: 59.6 g
- Fat: 3.2 g

Preparation time: 4 minutes
Cooking time: 10 minutes
Servings: 4

101. Chicken Florentine

INGREDIENTS

- 2 tsp olive oil
- 2 zucchinis, seeded, thinly sliced
- ½ cup green onion, sliced
- 2 chicken breasts, cubed
- ½ tsp salt
- ½ tsp thyme, ground
- 3 cups long-grain rice, cooked
- 4 cups fresh spinach, chopped
- ¼ cup Parmesan cheese, grated

DIRECTIONS

1. Heat the olive oil in a medium pot.
2. After 10 minutes, or till poultry is browned, add squash, onions, and chicken, turning regularly.
3. Salt, thyme, rice, and spinach should all be added at this point. Simmer, stir to combine, for a further 6-8 minutes, just until the spinach has wilted.
4. Take off the heat, pour into a large serving dish, and toss in the cheese. Serve.

NUTRITION

- Calories: 360
- Protein: 34 g
- Carbs: 18 g
- Fat: 23 g

Preparation time: 2 minutes
Cooking time: 11 minutes
Servings: 4

102. Chipotle Black Bean Chili

INGREDIENTS
- 1 tsp olive oil
- 1 cup onion, finely chopped
- Garlic cloves, minced
- ½ tsp chipotle powder
- ½ tsp cumin
- ¼ tsp salt
- 30 oz can of black beans, drained and rinsed
- 28 oz tomatoes, seeded and chopped
- 1 tsp fresh cilantro

DIRECTIONS
1. Warm the olive oil in a nonstick pan skillet over moderate heat.
2. Sauté for 5 minutes, or until onion and cloves of garlic are tender. Bring to a simmer with chipotle powder, cumin, pepper, beans, and tomatoes.
3. Turn off the heat, cover, and cook for 15–25 minutes, or until chili thickens.

NUTRITION
- Calories: 256
- Protein: 13 g
- Carbs: 47 g
- Fat: 3 g

Preparation time: 5 minutes
Cooking time: 2 minutes
Servings: 4

103. Garnish with Fresh Cilantro

INGREDIENTS
- ¾ cups cottage cheese
- ¼ cup carrots, shredded
- 2 tbsp. Green onion, sliced
- ½ cup tomatoes, seeded, chopped
- ½ cup cabbage, chopped
- 1 tsp lime juice
- 4 Whole wheat tortillas

DIRECTIONS
1. Combine the tomato, carrot, onion, cheese, and then cabbage in a large mixing dish and stir thoroughly. Lemon juice should be added.
2. Fill tortillas with the filling, roll them up, and serve.

NUTRITION
- Calories: 280
- Protein: 15 g
- Carbs: 27 g
- Fat: 3 g

Preparation time: 8 minutes
Cooking time: 3 minutes
Servings: 4

104. Couscous with Chicken

INGREDIENTS

- 4 tsp olive oil
- 1 lb chicken thighs, sliced into strips
- Onion, chopped
- Garlic cloves, minced
- 1 cup carrots, shredded
- 1 tsp smoked paprika
- 1 tsp cumin
- ⅛ tsp cinnamon
- ½ tsp salt
- 1 cup dried fruits, chopped
- 4 cups chicken broth
- 2 tsp butter
- 1 ½ cup. couscous
- ½ cup Italian parsley, chopped

DIRECTIONS

1. Heat the oil in a big, wide skillet over medium heat.
2. Sauté for 3-4 minutes to brown the chicken. Sprinkle with spices and salt, then green onions, garlic, and carrots. Cook for 6-8 minutes in the oven.
3. Toss the fruits, veggies, and 2 ½ cup stock in a bowl and stir. Bring to a boil. Bring to low heat, lid, and cook for 10 minutes.
4. 1 ½ cups stock, brought to a simmer in a different medium saucepan, then toss in couscous.
5. Take off the heat, cover, and set aside to cool for 5 minutes. With just a fork, mix the rice and serve with the chicken.

NUTRITION

- Calories: 117
- Protein: 10.2 g
- Carbs: 14.2 g
- Fat: 2.6 g

Preparation time: 4 minutes
Cooking time: 10 minutes
Servings: 4

105. Couscous with Vegetables

INGREDIENTS

- 1 ½ cup chicken broth
- 1 cup couscous
- 4 tsp olive oil, divided
- 1 Red onion, chopped
- 1 tbsp. Garlic cloves, minced
- 2 Tomatoes, seeded and chopped
- 1 Yellow bell pepper, seeded and chopped
- 1 Red bell pepper, seeded and chopped
- 1 Zucchinis, seeded and chopped
- 1 cup peas, thawed from froz en
- 2 tsp balsamic vinegar
- 2 tsp Feta cheese, crumbled

DIRECTIONS

1. Put chicken broth and 1 tbsp olive oil to a simmer in a medium pot over high temperature. Take the pan from the heat and mix in the couscous. Allow for 5-10 minutes of rest time after covering
2. Sauté the garlic and onions in a different skillet over medium heat with the excess oil.
3. Combine the tomatoes, bell peppers, and then zucchinis in a large mixing bowl. Simmer, occasionally stirring, until the veggies are soft.
4. Simmer for a further 2-3 minutes after adding the peas. Mix in the vinegar and cheese until well combined.
5. Place the veggie mixture on top of the couscous. Serve.

NUTRITION

- Calories: 219
- Protein: 6.5 g
- Carbs: 40.3 g
- Fat: 4 g

Preparation time: 15 minutes
Cooking time: 10 minutes
Servings: 4

106. Easy Beef Stir-Fry

INGREDIENTS

- ¼ cup orange juice
- ¼ cup low-sodium soy sauce
- 2 tsp rice vinegar
- ¼ cup water
- 2 tsp canola oil
- 8 oz beef round tip steak, thinly sliced
- Garlic cloves, minced
- 6 oz peas, thawed from froz en
- Bunch broccoli florets
- 8 oz edamame, shelled
- 1 ½ tsp cornstarch, dissolved in ¼ cup warm water

DIRECTIONS

1. Place the orange juice, soy sauce, rice vinegar, and water in a small mixing dish and stir gently.
2. 1 tsp canola oil, heated over moderate heat in a large nonstick skillet Sauté, occasionally tossing, for 2 minutes, or until the meat is slightly browned. Remove the steak from the pan and place it on a different platter.
3. Sauté garlic for 1 minute over a moderate flame without browning it in the other tsp oil. Sauté for 3 minutes with the peas, broccoli, and edamame.
4. Sauté, constantly stirring, for 5 minutes, or until the cauliflower is cooked and crisp-tender.
5. Return the cut beef to the skillet and mix the powdered cornstarch in water until all the ingredients are well combined.
6. Simmer until the steak is cooked through and the sauce has thickened somewhat. Right away, serve.

NUTRITION

- Calories: 219
- Protein: 6.5 g
- Carbs: 40.3 g
- Fat: 4 g

Preparation time: 10 minutes
Cooking time: 5 minutes
Servings: 4

107. Easy Turkey Chili

INGREDIENTS

- 3 tsp olive oil
- 1 tbsp. Garlic cloves, minced
- 1 Onion, chopped
- 1 lb ground turkey
- 2 Bay leaf
- 1 tsp ground cumin
- 1 tsp dried oregano
- 2 Tomato, seeded, chopped
- 14 oz can of tomato sauce
- 1 cup beef broth
- 1 tsp salt
- 28 oz can of red beans, rinsed

DIRECTIONS

1. In a large pot, heat oil over medium heat and cook garlic and onions for 5 minutes.
2. Increase heat to high and add turkey, bay leaf, cumin, and oregano. Cook until turkey has browned, about 5–7 minutes.
3. Add tomato, tomato sauce, broth, and salt. Bring the pot to a boil and then lower the heat to simmer. Cover and simmer for about 20 minutes.
4. Add beans and more water if needed and continue to simmer for 25 more minutes. Serve.

NUTRITION

- Calories: 373
- Protein: 29 g
- Carbs: 10 g
- Fat: 24 g

Preparation time: 5 minutes
Cooking time: 4 minutes
Servings: 4

108. Garbanzo Pita Pockets

INGREDIENTS

- 15 oz can of garbanzo beans, rinsed
- 6 oz can of artichokes, quartered, liquid reserved
- 1 tsp black olives. sliced
- 1 tsp green olives, sliced
- 1 Green bell pepper, seeded, chopped
- 1 Red bell pepper, seeded and chopped
- 1 Small red onion, thinly sliced
- 2 tsp red wine vinegar
- ½ cup fresh basil, chopped
- 4 Whole-wheat pita pockets

DIRECTIONS

1. Artichokes, Garbanzo beans and juice, olives, basil, peppers, onion, vinegar, and garlic should all be combined in a large mixing basin. Cast aside after mixing well.
2. To create a pouch, slice flatbread. Cover every pita with garbanzo mixture, starting with a cabbage leaf. Serve.

NUTRITION

- Calories: 373
- Protein: 29 g
- Carbs: 10 g
- Fat: 24 g

Preparation time: 4 minutes
Cooking time: 6 minutes
Servings: 4

109. Grilled Fish Tacos

INGREDIENTS

- ¼ tsp salt
- 1 Lemon, juiced
- 2 tsp olive oil
- 4 Fish filets, trout, or tilapia
- ½ cup red onion, chopped
- ½ cup jicama, peeled, chopped
- ⅓ cup red bell pepper, chopped
- ⅔ cup fresh cilantro, finely chopped
- 1 cup black beans, drained, rinsed
- 1 Lime, zest, and juice
- 1 tsp plain yogurt
- 4 Whole wheat tortillas

DIRECTIONS

1. Add salt, lemon juice, and olive oil to a mixing bowl. Spread the marinade over the cutlets and set aside for 10 minutes to marinate.
2. Fry the fish for 3 minutes at a high temperature.
3. When preparing a "salsa," mix beans, jicama, bell pepper, cilantro, onion, lemon zest and juice, and yogurt in a separate dish.
4. Arrange the fish on a warmed tortilla, top with "salsa," and divide it in 2. Serve.

NUTRITION

- Calories: 244
- Protein: 16 g
- Carbs: 18 g
- Fat: 12 g

Preparation time: 3 minutes
Cooking time: 4 minutes
Servings: 4

110. Grilled Steak with Spinach and Apple Salad

INGREDIENTS

- 4 Beef steaks, rib-eye, or sirloin
- 4 tsp olive oil
- Salt and pepper to taste
- 1 tsp balsamic vinegar
- 2 cups fresh baby spinach, washed and dried
- 1 Apple, unpeeled and sliced
- 4 oz Parmesan cheese, grated

DIRECTIONS

1. Arrange the steaks for the grilling by brushing them with 2 tsp oil and season them with salt and black pepper. Grilled to preferred medium-rare on high temperature, approximately 7 minutes each side for well. Place the steaks on a dish to cool and allow the juices to redistribute before cutting them.
2. To create the vinaigrette, mix up balsamic vinegarand 2 tsp oil, and season with salt and pepper in a mixing bowl.
3. Layer spinach, apples, and steak that has been sliced crosswise on separate dishes. Pour with vinaigrette and sprinkle with Parmesan cheese before serving

NUTRITION

- Calories: 244
- Protein: 16 g
- Carbs: 18 g
- Fat: 12 g

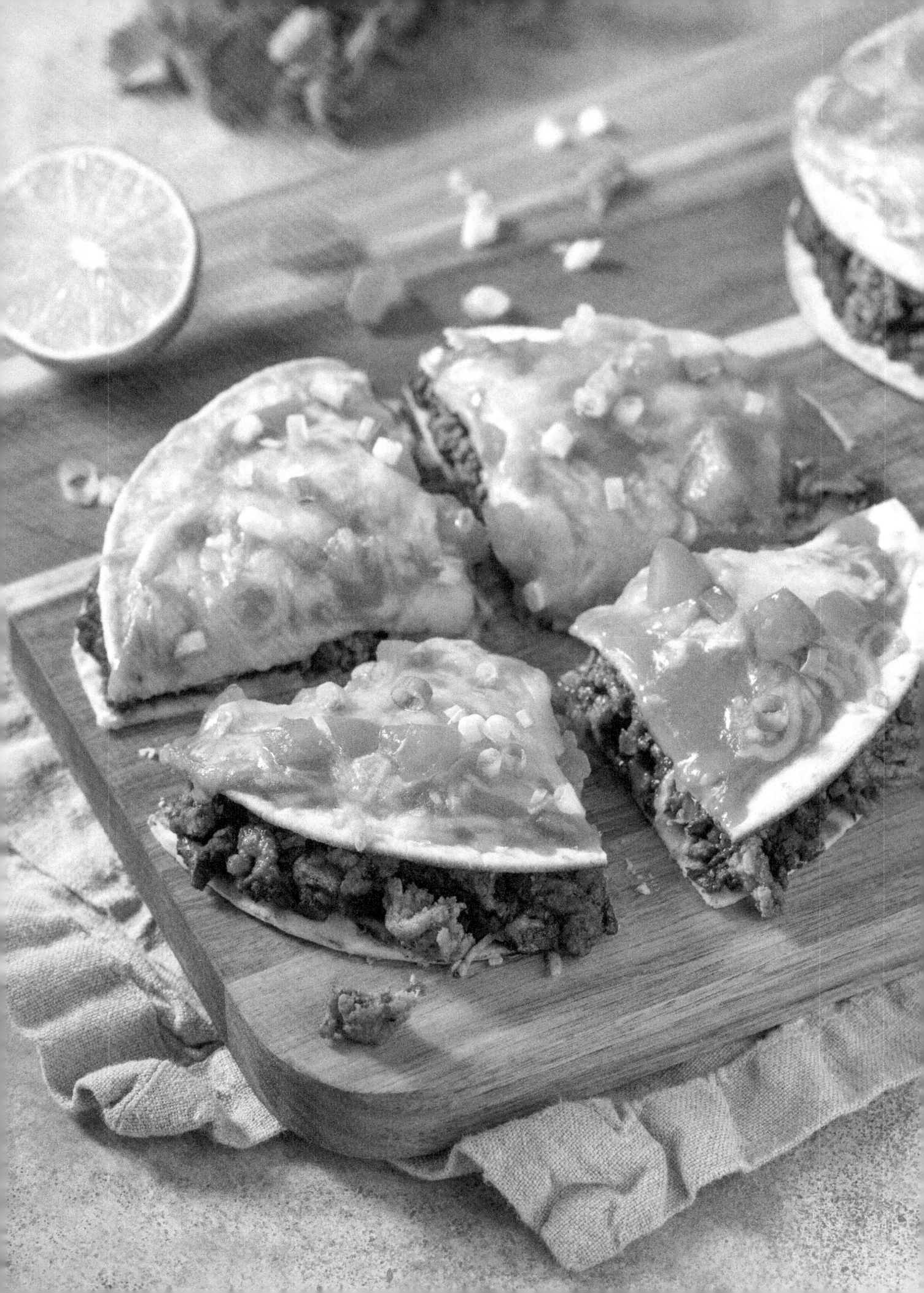

Chapter 12. High-Fiber Recipes

Preparation time: 20 minutes
Cooking time: 0 minutes
Servings: 4

111. Great Luncheon Salad

INGREDIENTS

For the salad:

- ½ cup homemade vegetable broth
- ½ cup couscous
- 3 cups canned red kidney beans, rinsed and drained
- 2 large tomatoes, peeled, seeded, and chopped
- 5 cups fresh spinach, torn

For the dressing:

- 1 garlic clove, minced
- 2 tbsp shallots, minced
- 2 tsp lemon zest, grated finely
- ¼ cup fresh lemon juice
- 2 tbsp extra-virgin olive oil
- Salt and freshly ground black pepper, to taste

DIRECTIONS

1. In a pan, add the broth over medium heat and bring to a boil.
2. Add the couscous and stir to combine.
3. Cover the pan and immediately remove it from the heat.
4. Set aside and covered for about 5-10 minutes or until all the liquid is absorbed.
5. For the salad: In a large serving bowl, add the couscous and remaining ingredients and stir to combine.
6. For the dressing: In another small bowl, add all the ingredients and beat until well combined.
7. Pour the dressing over the salad and gently toss to coat well.
8. Serve immediately.

NUTRITION

- Calories: 341
- Carbs: 53.2 g
- Protein: 15.7 g
- Fat: 8.5 g
- Sugar: 6.6 g
- Sodium: 670 mg
- Fiber: 13.5 g

Preparation time: 15 minutes
Cooking time: 5 minutes
Servings: 2

112. Flavors Powerhouse Lunch Meal

INGREDIENTS

- 1 large avocado
- 1¼ cup cooked chickpeas
- ¼ cup celery stalks, chopped
- 1 scallion (greed part), sliced
- 1 small garlic clove, minced
- 1½ tbsp fresh lemon juice
- ½ tsp olive oil
- Salt and freshly ground black pepper to taste
- 1 tbsp fresh cilantro, chopped

DIRECTIONS

1. Cut the avocado in half and then remove the pit.
2. With a spoon, scoop out the flesh from each avocado half.
3. Then, cut half of the avocado flesh into equal-sized cubes.
4. In a large bowl, add avocado cubes and remaining ingredients except for sunflower seeds and cilantro and toss to coat well.
5. Stuff each avocado half with chickpeas mixture evenly.
6. Serve immediately with the garnishing of cilantro.

NUTRITION

- Calories: 403
- Carbs: 0 g
- Protein: 9.8 g
- Fat: 22.6 g
- Sugar: 1.1 g
- Sodium: 546 mg
- Fiber: 13.8 g

Preparation time: 20 minutes
Cooking time: 40 minutes
Servings: 2

113. Eye-Catching Sweet Potato Boats

INGREDIENTS

For the sweet potatoes:
- 1 large sweet potato, halved lengthwise
- ½ tbsp olive oil
- Salt and freshly ground black pepper, to taste

For the filling:
- ½ tbsp olive oil
- ⅓ cup canned chickpeas, rinsed and drained
- 1 tsp curry powder
- ⅛ tsp garlic powder
- ⅓ cup cooked quinoa
- Salt and freshly ground black pepper, to taste
- 1 tsp fresh lime juice
- 1 tsp fresh cilantro, chopped

DIRECTIONS

1. Preheat the oven to 375°F.
2. Rub each sweet potato half with oil evenly.
3. Arrange the sweet potato halves onto a baking sheet, cut side down, and sprinkle with salt and black pepper.
4. Bake for about 40 minutes or until sweet potato becomes tender.
5. Meanwhile, for filling: In a skillet, heat the oil over medium heat and cook the chickpeas, curry powder, and garlic powder for about 6–8 minutes, stirring frequently.
6. Stir in the cooked quinoa, salt, and black pepper and remove from the heat.
7. Remove from the oven and arrange each sweet potato halves onto a plate.
8. With a fork, fluff the flesh of each half slightly.
9. Place chickpeas mixture in each half and drizzle with lime juice
10. Serve immediately with the garnishing of cilantro and sesame seeds.

NUTRITION

- Calories: 286
- Carbs: 43 g
- Protein: 8.2 g
- Fat: 9.7 g
- Sugar: 6.6 g
- Sodium: 175 mg
- Fiber: 8 g

Preparation time: 15 minutes
Cooking time: 20 minutes
Servings: 8

114. Mexican Enchiladas

INGREDIENTS

- 1 (14 oz) can of red beans, drained, rinsed, and mashed
- 2 cups cheddar cheese, grated
- 2 cups tomato sauce
- ½ cup onion, chopped
- ¼ cup black olives, pitted and sliced
- 2 tsp garlic salt
- 8 whole-wheat tortillas

DIRECTIONS

1. Preheat the oven to 350°F.
2. In a medium bowl, add the mashed beans, cheese, 1 cup tomato sauce, onions, olives, and garlic salt, and mix well.
3. Place about ⅓ cup of the bean mixture along the center of each tortilla.
4. Roll up each tortilla and place enchiladas in a large baking dish.
5. Place the remaining tomato sauce on top of the filled tortillas.
6. Bake for about 15–20 minutes.
7. Serve warm.

NUTRITION

- Calories: 358
- Carbs: 46.2 g
- Protein: 20.6 g
- Fat: 11.2 g
- Sugar: 4.5 g
- Sodium: 550 mg
- Fiber: 10.3 g

Preparation time: 15 minutes
Cooking time: 15 minutes
Servings: 3

115. Unique Banana Curry

INGREDIENTS

- 2 tbsp olive oil
- 2 yellow onions, chopped
- 8 garlic cloves, minced
- 2 tbsp curry powder
- 1 tbsp ground ginger
- 1 tbsp ground cumin
- 1 tsp ground turmeric
- 1 tsp ground cinnamon
- 1 tsp red chili powder
- Salt and freshly ground black pepper, to taste
- ⅓ cup plain yogurt
- 1 cup tomato puree
- 2 bananas, peeled and sliced
- 3 tomatoes, peeled, seeded, and chopped finely

DIRECTIONS

1. In a large pan, heat the oil over medium heat and sauté the onion for about 4–5 minutes.
2. Add garlic, curry powder and spices, and sauté for about 1 minute.
3. Add the yogurt and tomato sauce and bring to a gentle boil.
4. Stir in the bananas and simmer for about 3 minutes.
5. Stir in the tomatoes and simmer for about 1–2 minutes.
6. Remove from the heat and serve hot.

NUTRITION

- Calories: 318
- Carbs: 49.7 g
- Protein: 9 g
- Fat: 12.2 g
- Sugar: 24.2 g
- Sodium: 138 mg
- Fiber: 9.5 g

Preparation time: 10 minutes
Cooking time: 30 minutes
Servings: 4

116. Vegan-Friendly Platter

INGREDIENTS

- 1 tbsp olive oil
- 2 small onions, chopped
- 5 garlic cloves, chopped finely
- 1 tsp dried oregano
- 1 tsp ground cumin
- ½ tsp ground ginger
- Salt and freshly ground black pepper, to taste
- 2 cups tomatoes, peeled, seeded, and chopped
- 2 (13 ½ oz) cans of black beans, rinsed and drained
- ½ cup homemade vegetable broth

DIRECTIONS

1. In a pan, heat the olive oil over medium heat and cook the onion for about 5-7 minutes, stirring frequently.
2. Add the garlic, oregano, spices, salt, and black pepper and cook for about 1 minute.
3. Add the tomatoes and cook for about 1-2 minutes.
4. Add in the beans and broth and bring to a boil.
5. Reduce the heat to medium-low and simmer, covered for about 15 minutes.
6. Serve hot.

NUTRITION

- Calories: 327
- Carbs: 54.1 g
- Protein: 19.1 g
- Fat: 5.1 g
- Sugar: 4 g
- Sodium: 595 mg
- Fiber: 18.8 g

Preparation time: 15 minutes
Cooking time: 15 minutes
Servings: 4

117. Armenian Style Chickpeas

INGREDIENTS

- 2 tbsp olive oil
- 1 medium yellow onion, chopped
- 4 garlic cloves, minced
- 1 tsp dried thyme, crushed
- 1 tsp dried oregano, crushed
- ½ tsp paprika
- 1 cup tomato, chopped finely
- 2 ½ cup canned chickpeas, rinsed and drained
- 5 cups Swiss chard, chopped
- 2 tbsp water
- 2 tbsp fresh lemon juice
- Salt and freshly ground black pepper to taste
- 3 tbsp fresh basil, chopped

DIRECTIONS

1. In a skillet, heat the olive oil over medium heat and sauté the onion for about 6-8 minutes.
2. Add garlic, herbs and paprika, and sauté for about 1 minute.
3. Add the Swiss chard and 2 tbsp water and cook for about 2-3 minutes.
4. Add the tomatoes and chickpeas and cook for about 2-3 minutes.
5. Add in the lemon juice, salt and black pepper, and remove from the heat.
6. Serve hot with the garnishing of basil.

NUTRITION

- Calories: 260
- Carbs: 34 g
- Protein: 12 g
- Fat: 8.6 g
- Sugar: 3.1 g
- Sodium: 178 mg
- Fiber: 9 g

Preparation time: 15 minutes
Cooking time: 1 hour 10 minutes
Servings: 8

118. Protein-Packed Soup

INGREDIENTS
- 2 tbsp olive oil
- 1½ lb ground turkey
- Salt and freshly ground black pepper, to taste
- 1 large carrot, peeled and chopped
- 1 large celery stalk, chopped
- 1 large onion, chopped
- 6 garlic cloves, chopped
- 1 tsp dried rosemary
- 1 tsp dried oregano
- 2 large potatoes, peeled and chopped
- 8-9 cup chicken bone broth
- 4-5 cups tomatoes, peeled, seeded, and chopped
- 2 cups dry lentils
- ¼ cup fresh parsley, chopped

DIRECTIONS
1. In a large soup pan, heat the olive oil over medium-high heat and cook the turkey for about 5 minutes or until browned.
2. With a slotted spoon, transfer the turkey into a bowl and set it aside.
3. In the same pan, add the carrot, celery, onion, garlic, and dried herbs over medium heat and cook for about 5 minutes.
4. Add the potatoes and cook for about 4-5 minutes.
5. Add the cooked turkey, tomatoes, and broth and bring to a boil over high heat.
6. Reduce the heat to low and cook, covered for about 10 minutes.
7. Add the lentils and cook, covered for about 40 minutes.
8. Stir in black pepper and remove from the heat.
9. Serve hot with the garnishing of parsley.

NUTRITION
- Calories: 485
- Carbs: 44.6 g
- Protein: 43 g
- Fat: 16.5 g
- Sugar: 8.5 g
- Sodium: 452 mg
- Fiber: 16.6 g

Preparation time: 15 minutes
Cooking time: 50 minutes
Servings: 4

119. One-Pot Dinner Soup

INGREDIENTS
- 1 tbsp olive oil
- 1 cup yellow onion, chopped
- ½ cup carrots, peeled and chopped
- ½ cup celery, chopped
- 2 garlic cloves, minced
- 4 cups homemade vegetable broth
- 2 ½ cup sweet potatoes, peeled and chopped
- 1 cup red lentils, rinsed
- 1 ½ tbsp fresh lemon juice
- Salt and freshly ground black pepper, to taste
- 2 tbsp fresh cilantro, chopped

DIRECTIONS
1. In a large Dutch oven, heat the oil over medium heat and sauté the onion, carrot, and celery for about 5-7 minutes.
2. Add the garlic and sauté for about 1 minute.
3. Add the sweet potatoes and cook for about 1-2 minutes.
4. Add in the broth and bring to a boil.
5. Reduce the heat to low and simmer, covered for about 5 minutes.
6. Stir in the red lentils and gain bring to a boil over medium-high heat.
7. Reduce the heat to low and simmer, covered for about 25-30 minutes or until desired doneness.
8. Stir in the lemon juice, salt, and black pepper and remove from the heat.
9. Serve hot with the garnishing of cilantro.

NUTRITION
- Calories: 471
- Carbs: 61 g
- Protein: 19.3 g
- Fat: 5.6 g
- Sugar: 4.4 g
- Sodium: 836 mg
- Fiber: 19.7 g

Preparation time: 15 minutes
Cooking time: 45 minutes

120. 3-Beans Soup

INGREDIENTS

- ¼ cup olive oil
- 1 large onion, chopped
- 1 large sweet potato, peeled and cubed
- 3 carrots, peeled and chopped
- 3 celery stalks, chopped
- 3 garlic cloves, minced
- 2 tsp dried thyme, crushed
- 1 tbsp red chili powder
- 1 tbsp ground cumin
- 4 large tomatoes, peeled, seeded, and chopped finely
- 2 (16 oz) cans of Great Northern beans, rinsed and drained
- 2 (15 ¼ oz) cans of red kidney beans, rinsed and drained
- 1 (15 oz) can of black beans, drained and rinsed
- 12 cups of homemade vegetable broth
- 1 cup fresh cilantro, chopped
- Salt and freshly ground black pepper, to taste

DIRECTIONS

1. In a Dutch oven, heat the oil over medium heat and sauté the onion, sweet potato, carrot, and celery for about 6–8 minutes.
2. Add the garlic, thyme, chili powder, and cumin and sauté for about 1 minute.
3. Add in the tomatoes and cook for about 2–3 minutes.
4. Add the beans and broth and bring to a boil over medium-high heat.
5. Cover the pan with the lid and cook for about 25–30 minutes.
6. Stir in the cilantro and remove from heat.
7. Serve hot.

NUTRITION

- Calories: 411
- Carbs: 69.7 g
- Protein: 22.7 g
- Fat: 5.7 g
- Sugar: 7.1 g
- Sodium: 931 mg
- Fiber: 18.9 g

Preparation time: 20 minutes
Cooking time: 30 minutes
Servings: 4

121. Pork and Penne Pasta

INGREDIENTS

- 1 lb whole-wheat penne pasta
- 1 lb ground pork lean
- 2 tbsp extra-virgin olive oil
- 1 small onion, chopped
- 2 garlic cloves, minced
- 1 (15 oz) can of tomatoes, diced and seeded
- 2 cups green zucchini, sliced into ¼-inch cubes
- 8 oz baby spinach, fresh and chopped
- 1 cup low-fat Parmesan cheese, grated

DIRECTIONS

1. Bring a pot of water to a boil, and ensure that the water is salted. Cook the pasta to an al dente consistency or according to package directions.
2. In a non-stick pan, cook the ground pork over medium heat for 8 minutes or until it is browned, ensure to break up any large pieces in the pan.
3. Remove pork and set it aside. Discard drippings. Add in your oil on medium heat.
4. Cook onions and garlic for about 5 minutes or until soft. Add tomatoes and zucchini and continue cooking for 5 minutes more.
5. Add spinach and cook until it just wilts, 2–3 minutes. Place the pork back into the skillet and add ½ cup cheese; stir and heat through.
6. Plate your pasta then tops with your meat mixture. Toss well and top evenly with cheese.

NUTRITION

- Calories: 206
- Fat: 9 g
- Carbs: 24 g
- Fiber: 13 g
- Protein: 17 g

Preparation time: 10 minutes
Cooking time: 0 minutes
Servings: 4

122. Chicken and Quinoa Pita

INGREDIENTS

- 1 cup fat-free cream cheese, softened
- 1 tbsp fat-free mayonnaise
- 2 cups cooked chicken, cubed
- 1 cup tomatoes, seeded and sliced
- 1 (14 oz) can of quinoa, cooked
- 4 Romaine lettuce leaves
- 2 cups alfalfa sprouts, rinsed and drained
- 4 whole-wheat pita bread, round

DIRECTIONS

1. In a bowl, combine mayonnaise and cream cheese until it is fully mixed. Add chicken, tomatoes, and quinoa; mix well. Slice the pita bread to form a pocket. Fill your pitas with lettuce and chicken. Top with alfalfa sprouts. Serve.

NUTRITION

- Calories: 331
- Fat: 23 g
- Carbs: 5 g
- Fiber: 2 g
- Protein: 26 g

Preparation time: 15 minutes
Cooking time: 18 minutes
Servings: 4

123. Turkey Florentine

INGREDIENTS

- 2 tbsp olive oil
- 2 medium zucchinis, seeded and thinly sliced
- ½ cup green onions, sliced
- 2 cups turkey breast, cubed
- ½ tsp salt
- ½ tsp thyme, ground
- 2 tbsp pimento, chopped
- 3 cups cooked long-grain rice
- 4 cups fresh baby spinach
- ¼ cup low-fat Parmesan cheese, freshly grated

DIRECTIONS

1. In a non-stick pan, heat olive oil over moderate heat. Add zucchini, turkey, and onions, and stir every now and then for 5–10 minutes.
2. Add salt, thyme, pimento, rice, and spinach. Cook and stir for another 6–8 minutes or until heated through and spinach wilts.
3. Remove from heat, transfer to a large serving bowl, and stir in cheese. Serve.

NUTRITION

- Calories: 593
- Fat: 8 g
- Carbs: 11 g
- Fiber: 4 g
- Protein: 12 g

124. Chicken Lettuce Wraps

Preparation time: 15 minutes
Cooking time: 0 minutes
Servings: 2

INGREDIENTS

- ¼ cup low-fat mayonnaise
- 2 tsp lemon juice
- ½ cup white beans, canned, cooked, and drained
- ⅓ cup crumbled Feta cheese
- 2 tbsp chopped pimentos
- 8 large lettuce leaves, washed and dried
- ½ lb chicken breast strips, cooked (preferably grilled)

DIRECTIONS

1. In a medium bowl, combine mayonnaise and lemon juice. Stir in beans, mashing slightly with a fork.
2. Add cheese and pimentos and mix lightly. Spread lettuce leaves evenly with bean mixture.
3. Top with chicken; roll-up. Serve.

NUTRITION

- Calories: 338
- Fat: 10 g
- Carbs: 39 g
- Fiber: 9 g
- Protein: 26 g

---

125. Couscous with Turkey

Preparation time: 20 minutes
Cooking time: 26 minutes
Servings: 4

INGREDIENTS

- 4 tbsp extra-virgin olive oil
- 1 lb turkey thighs, boneless, skinless, and chopped
- 1 chopped onion
- 3 minced garlic cloves
- 1 cup shredded carrots
- 1 tsp smoked paprika
- ⅛ tsp ground cinnamon
- ½ tsp salt
- 1 cup dried fruits, chopped, pitted dates, and apricots
- 4 cups turkey stock, divided
- 2 tbsp butter
- 1 ½ cups couscous
- ½ cup chopped Italian parsley

DIRECTIONS

1. Set your oil to get hot on medium heat. Cook turkey and brown for 3–4 minutes on each side.
2. Add onions, garlic, carrots, and season with spices and salt. Cook 6–8 minutes.
3. Stir the fruits into the turkey and vegetables, and 2 ½ cup stock.
4. Allow boiling. Turn down the heat to low, cover, and let it simmer for 10 minutes.
5. In a separate small saucepan, over medium heat, pour 1 ½ cup stock and bring up to a boil then stir in the couscous.
6. Take the content off the heat and let it stand 5 minutes while the cover is on. Fluff with a fork and serve with turkey.

NUTRITION

- Calories: 469
- Fat: 24 g
- Carbs: 40 g
- Fiber: 4 g
- Protein: 18 g

Preparation time: 15 minutes
Cooking time: 17 minutes
Servings: 4

126. Ham, Bean, and Cabbage Stew

INGREDIENTS

- 1 tbsp extra-virgin olive oil
- 8 oz chopped smoked ham
- 1 chopped large onion
- 2 sliced celery stalks
- 5 garlic cloves, chopped finely
- 4 cups chicken broth
- 1 (28 oz) can of tomatoes, seedless and drained
- 3 cups whole-wheat pasta
- 8 oz coleslaw
- 2 (14 oz) cans of kidney beans
- 1 tsp dried basil
- 1 tsp dried rosemary

DIRECTIONS

1. In a good size pot, heat olive oil over medium heat. Cook ham, onion, celery, and garlic stirring occasionally, until vegetables are tender.
2. Stir in broth and tomatoes, breaking up tomatoes. Stir the pasta in, heat to boiling, and turn down the heat low.
3. Cover and simmer for about 10 minutes or until pasta is tender. Stir in coleslaw, beans, basil, and oregano.
4. Bring stew to a boil and reduce heat to low. Simmer uncovered for about 5–7 minutes or until cabbage is tender.

NUTRITION

- Calories: 543
- Fat: 21 g
- Carbs: 47 g
- Fiber: 8 g
- Protein: 40 g

Snack and desserts recipes

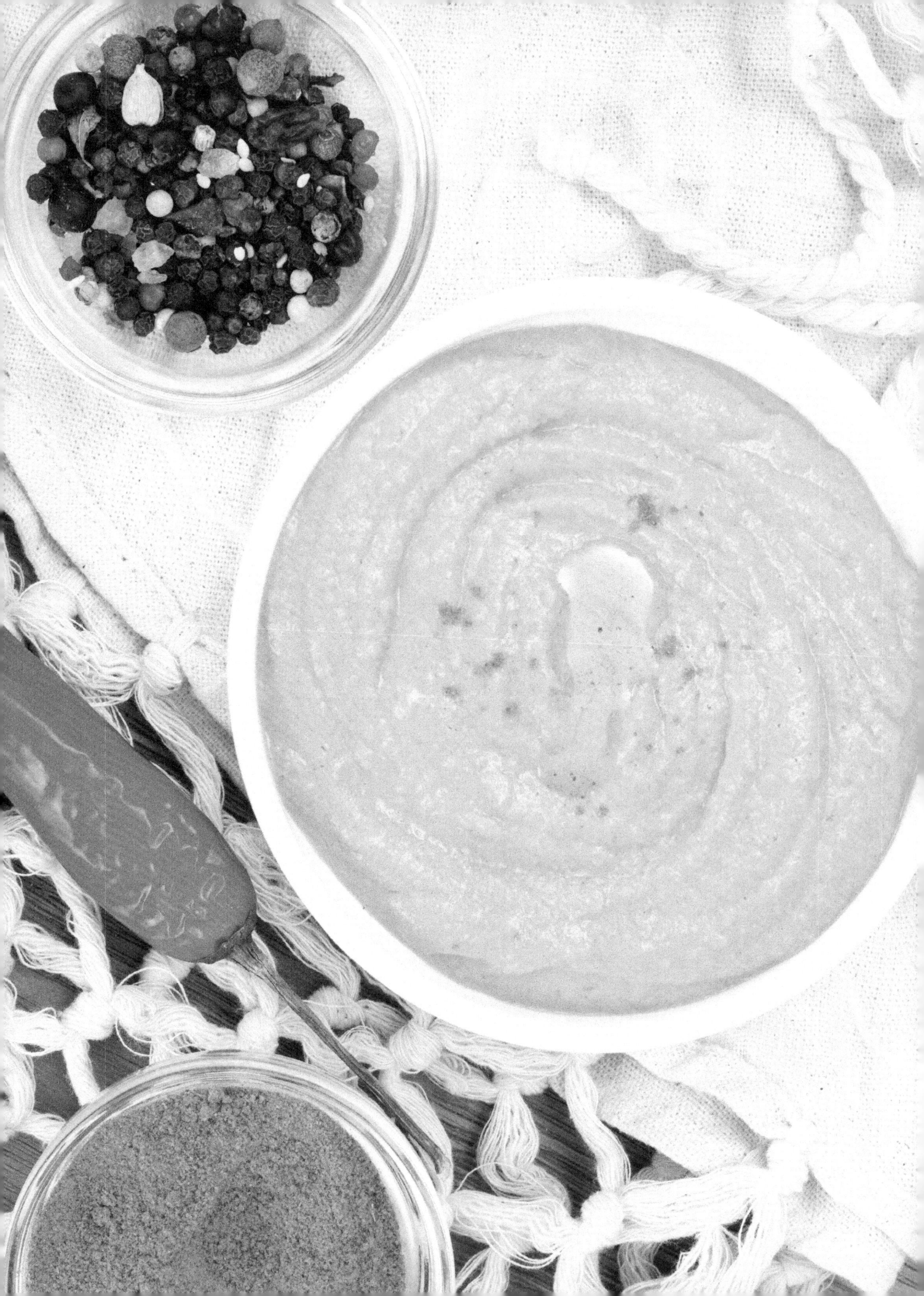

Chapter 13. Clear Liquid Recipes

Preparation time: 10 minutes
Cooking time: 0 minutes
Servings: 4

127. Hummus with Tahini and Turmeric

INGREDIENTS

- 2 cans of chickpeas, drained
- 50 ml lemon juice
- 60 ml tahini
- 1 garlic clove, minced
- 2 tbsp extra-virgin olive oil
- ½ tbsp turmeric powder
- ½ teaspoon sea salt

DIRECTIONS

1. Mix the tahini and lemon juice with olive oil, garlic, turmeric, and salt for about 30 seconds using a hand blender or kitchen utensil.
2. Add the chickpeas and puree, making sure that no chickpeas remain unmixed on the sides. Pound until a uniform mixture is obtained.
3. Garnish with paprika powder and enjoy with any snacks, such as vegetable sticks.

NUTRITION

- Calories: 33
- Carbs: 8.1 g
- Protein: 0.2 g
- Fat: 0.1 g
- Sugar: 7.6 g
- Sodium: 130 mg
- Fiber: 0.1 g

Preparation time: 10 minutes
Cooking time: 15 minutes
Servings: 4

128. Fiber Bars

INGREDIENTS

- 120 g dried dates
- 120 g nuts (cashew, hazel, walnuts)

DIRECTIONS

1. Remove the date kernels and mash the fruits with a fork.
2. Chop the nuts in a blender, but they must not get the consistency of flour.
3. Mix the 2 together.
4. Form small "snakes" and flatten them lightly with a fork so that they get the shape of a bar.

NUTRITION

- Calories: 140
- Carbs: 0.6 g
- Protein: 25 g
- Fat: 2.6 g
- Sugar: 0.1 g
- Sodium: 73 mg

Preparation time: 10 minutes
Cooking time: 25–30 minutes
Servings: 4

129. Roasted Carrot Sticks in a Honey Garlic Marinade

INGREDIENTS

- 1 bunch of carrots, halved lengthways
- 2 garlic cloves, minced
- 1 tbsp honey
- 1 tbsp lemon juice (alternatively apple cider vinegar)
- 40 g butter
- 3 tbsp parsley, chopped

DIRECTIONS

1. Place the halved cst, melt the butter. Add the garlic, honey, and lemon/vinegar, and mix well.
2. Set over the carrots so that they are all covered with the marinade.
3. Bake in the oven at 180°C for about 25–30 minutes. Turn regularly.
4. Garnish with parsley and serve with herb quark or yogurt.

NUTRITION

- Calories: 216
- Fat: 1 g
- Carbs: 37 g
- Fiber: 4 g
- Protein: 8 g

Preparation time: 10 minutes
Cooking time: 5 minutes
Servings: 4

130. Apple and Pistachio Salad on Spinach

INGREDIENTS

- 1 ½ tbsp butter
- 1 pack of baby spinach
- 1 apple, diced small
- 1 tsp ginger, grated
- 60 g pistachios
- 1 tbsp mustard
- 40 g ricotta cheese
- 1 tbsp honey
- 1 tbsp lemon juice
- Salt and pepper

DIRECTIONS

1. Dissolve the butter in the pan, and add the apple pieces, honey, ginger, and mustard. Fry over medium heat until the apples are lightly caramelized (about 3–5 minutes).
2. Wash the spinach and divide between 2 bowls. Place the apples on the salad, garnish with Ricotta, and season with a little lemon juice, pistachios, salt, and pepper as desired.

NUTRITION

- Calories: 37
- Fat: 1 g
- Carbs: 3 g
- Fiber: 0 g
- Protein: 4 g
- Sodium: 58 mg

Preparation time: 10 minutes
Cooking time: 0 minutes
Servings: 4

131. Tomato Cashew Pesto

INGREDIENTS
- 95 g dried tomatoes
- 50 g cashew nuts
- 2 garlic cloves, minced
- 5 tbsp extra-virgin olive oil
- 1 tbsp oregano
- Parmesan cheese (optional)
- Salt and pepper to taste

DIRECTIONS
1. Puree the garlic, tomatoes, oregano, oil, and cashews with a hand blender until the mixture is even.
2. Mix with whole-wheat pasta and serve. Flavor to taste with salt and pepper then garnish with Parmesan.

NUTRITION
- Calories: 29
- Fat: 1 g
- Carbs: 2 g
- Fiber: 1 g
- Protein: 1 g

Preparation time: 10 minutes
Cooking time: 35 minutes
Servings: 4

132. Sweet Potato Aioli

INGREDIENTS
- 1 sweet potato
- 3 tbsp olive oil
- 1 tbsp mayonnaise
- 2-3 garlic cloves
- 1 tbsp parsley, chopped

DIRECTIONS
1. Bake the sweet potato in the oven until it is soft (about 35 minutes at 200°C).
2. Set out of the oven, let cool down briefly, peel and mix with 1 tablespoon of mayonnaise, oil, garlic, and parsley (use a hand blender).

NUTRITION
- Calories: 75
- Carbs: 0.1 g
- Protein: 13.4 g
- Fat: 1.7 g
- Sugar: 0 g
- Sodium: 253 mg

Preparation time: 10 minutes
Cooking time: 25 minutes
Servings: 4

133. Eggplant Paste

INGREDIENTS

- 1 eggplant
- 2 tbsp tahini
- 2 garlic cloves
- 1 tbsp lemon juice
- A pinch of turmeric
- 30 g black olives
- 1 tbsp olive oil
- 1 tbsp parsley, chopped
- Salt and pepper to taste

DIRECTIONS

1. Grill the eggplant in the oven at 190°C for at least 20 minutes (until it is soft!).
2. Let cool and remove the skin. Set the eggplant in a container and use a fork to mash the meat into a paste.
3. Add the tahini, garlic, turmeric, olives, olive oil, and lemon juice; mix well. Season to taste with salt and pepper.
4. Garnish with parsley.

NUTRITION

- Calories: 75
- Carbs: 0.1 g
- Protein: 13.4 g
- Fat: 1.7 g
- Sugar: 0 g
- Sodium: 253 mg

Preparation time: 10 minutes
Cooking time: 5 minutes
Servings: 4

134. Catalan Style Spinach

INGREDIENTS

- 200 g fresh spinach
- 2 garlic cloves
- 2 tbsp cashew nuts
- 3 tbsp raisins
- 2-3 tbsp extra-virgin olive oil

DIRECTIONS

1. Warm the oil and fry the garlic over medium heat.
2. After 1-2 minutes add the cashews and raisins. Fry for another minute.
3. Add the spinach (do not boil!), and stir well.
4. Serve with Goat cheese and whole meal baguette.

NUTRITION

- Calories: 59
- Fat: 1 g
- Carbs: 14 g
- Fiber: 1 g
- Protein: 1 g
- Sodium: 304 mg

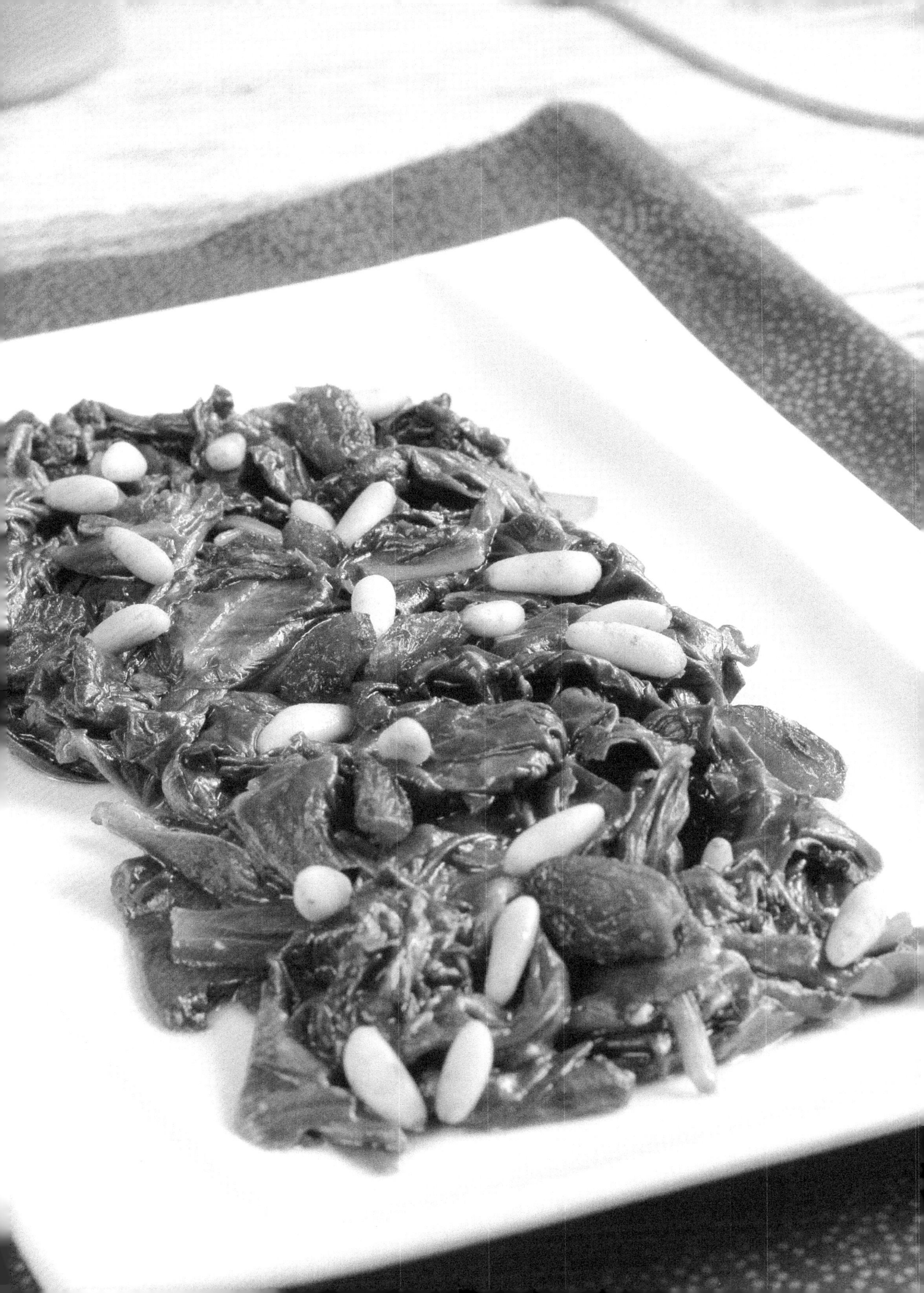

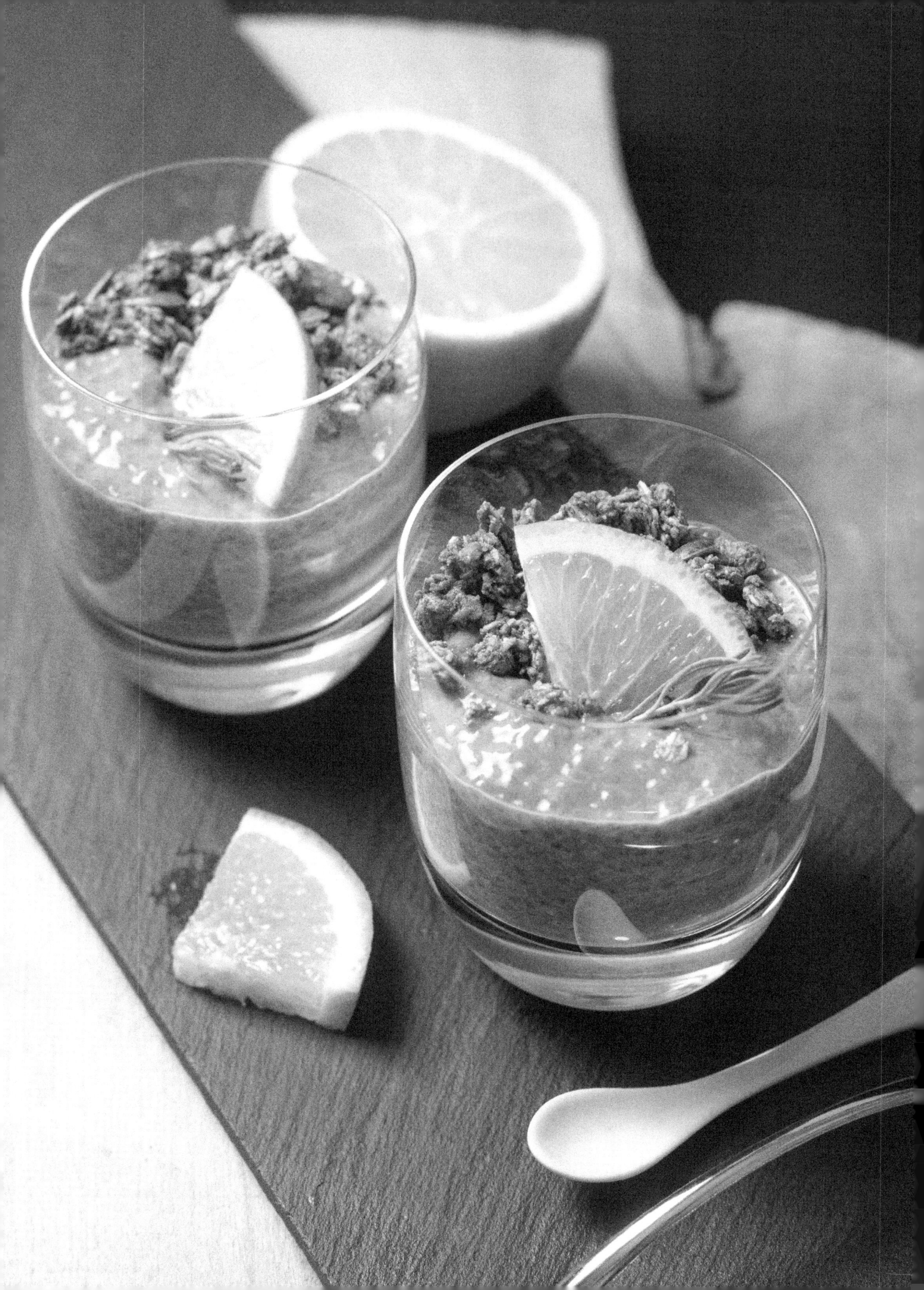

Chapter 14. Low-Residue Recipes

Preparation time: 20 minutes
Cooking time: 1 hour
Servings: 5

135. Thai Coconut Lime Soup

INGREDIENTS
- 1 tbsp olive oil
- 2 small zucchini, chopped
- 1 red bell pepper, chopped
- 4 carrots, chopped
- 1 potato, washed and chopped
- 1 lime juice
- ¼ cup chives, chopped
- 2 tsp ground ginger
- 2 cans of lite coconut milk
- 3 tbsp low-sodium tamari
- ¼ tsp black pepper
- 4 cups vegetable stock
- Fresh basil for garnish, optional

DIRECTIONS
1. In a medium saucepan, heat the olive oil over medium heat. Cook for 2-3 minutes, until the zucchini, carrots, bell pepper, and potato are slightly cooked.
2. In a large bowl, combine the lime zest, lime juice, coconut milk, chives, ginger, ginger, tamari, and broth. Bring the soup to a boil over high heat, stirring constantly. Reduce the heat to low and let the soup simmer for 10–15 minutes after reaching a boil.
3. To serve, serve as is or over brown jasmine rice and cauliflower rice garnished with fresh basil.

NUTRITION
- Calories: 220
- Fat: 11 g
- Protein: 5 g
- Carbs: 28 g

Preparation time: 15 minutes
Cooking time: 45 minutes
Servings: 6

136. Low-FODMAP French Oven Beef Stew

INGREDIENTS
- 1 lb beef for stew
- 1 cup fennel bulb, diced
- 1 medium celery stalk
- 6 medium carrots
- 4 medium parsnips
- 4 medium potatoes
- ¼ cup tapioca quick cooking
- 1 cup tomato juice
- 1 tbsp sugar (optional)
- ½ tsp salt
- ½ tsp freshly ground pepper
- 1 tsp ground basil

DIRECTIONS
1. Preheat the oven to 300°F. Cut the meat into 4 cm (12-inch) pieces.
2. All vegetables should be well cleaned. Remove dirt from the potato skins by rubbing them. Celery stalks and fennel bulb cut into medium dice Carrots, parsnips and potatoes should be cut into medium pieces.
3. Combine all the ingredients in a mixing bowl. Except for the potatoes, which should be baked in a large oven-safe dish with a lid. Cover and bake for 3 hours in the oven.
4. Add the potatoes and bake for another hour. Enjoy.

NUTRITION
- Calories: 228
- Fat: 16 g
- Protein: 5 g
- Carbs: 25 g

Preparation time: 10 minutes
Cooking time: 45 minutes
Servings: 14

137. Veggie-Packed Low-FODMAP Soup

INGREDIENTS

- 1 tbsp olive oil
- 3 tsp smoked paprika
- 2 tsp cumin
- 1 ½ tsp chili powder
- 6 medium-large carrots sliced
- ¼ cup water
- 10 cup water
- 15 oz can of diced tomatoes, salt-free
- 6 oz can of tomato paste, salt-free
- 3 tbsp soy sauce or tamari, low-sodium
- 3 tbsp lemon juice
- 1 tbsp pure maple syrup
- 1 tsp salt
- Black pepper to taste
- 1 cup uncooked quinoa
- 6 cups collard greens, loosely packed, big stems removed

DIRECTIONS

1. In a large frying pan, pour the oil.
2. Combine the paprika, cumin, and chili powder in a bowl.
3. Increase heat to medium. Combine the sliced carrots, chopped tomatoes, tomato paste, and ¼ cup of water in a large bowl.
4. Cover the saucepan with a lid and simmer for 10 minutes, stirring regularly. If necessary, lower the heat.
5. While those ingredients are cooking, rinse the quinoa in a fine-mesh strainer under running cold water for 30–45 seconds and remove the large stems from the leaves.
6. Add the remaining ingredients to the pan and stir to combine.
7. Increase the heat to medium-high.
8. Bring the soup to a simmer with the lid on (about 8 minutes).
9. Reduce heat to medium.
10. Simmer for 30–35 minutes after removing the lid.

NUTRITION

- Calories: 98
- Fat: 1 g
- Protein: 20 g
- Carbs: 4 g

Preparation time: 5 minutes
Cooking time: 45 minutes
Servings: 1

138. Cranberry Almond Oatmeal

INGREDIENTS

- ½ cup rolled oats
- ½ cup lactose-free milk
- ½ cup water
- 1 tbsp creamy almond butter
- ¼ tsp ground cinnamon
- 2 tbsp cranberry sauce

DIRECTIONS

1. Prepare the rolled oats according to package directions by combining the oats, milk, and water. Stir in the almond butter and cinnamon when the oatmeal is done.
2. Serve with cranberry sauce on top.

NUTRITION

- Calories: 260
- Fat: 22 g
- Protein: 5 g
- Carbs: 25 g

Preparation time: 5 minutes
Cooking time: 30 minutes
Servings: 1

139. Quick Banana Bread Oatmeal

INGREDIENTS

- ⅓ ripe banana
- ¼ cup Bob's red mill gluten-free quick oats
- 3 tbsp quinoa flakes
- ¾ cup almond milk unsweetened vanilla
- ¼ tsp ground cinnamon
- 1 tbsp chopped walnuts
- ½ tbsp mini chocolate chips Enjoy Life, dairy-free (optional)

DIRECTIONS

1. Using a fork, mash the banana in a microwave-safe bowl. Combine quick oats, almond milk, quinoa flakes, and cinnamon in a bowl. Stir well.
2. Microwave on full power for 1 minute, stirring halfway through. Microwave for another 30 seconds or until the oats are cooked through.
3. Add the walnuts and mix well. If desired, top with chocolate chips. Enjoy.

NUTRITION

- Calories: 240
- Fat: 3 g
- Protein: 5 g
- Carbs: 26 g

Preparation time: 30 minutes
Cooking time: 1 hour 30 minutes
Servings: 4

140. Spicy Lemon Pasta with Shrimp

INGREDIENTS

- 1 (8-oz) box of gluten-free linguini
- 1 tbsp garlic olive oil infused
- 4 tbsp butter
- 1–1 ¼ lb uncooked large shrimp, peeled and deveined
- 1 tsp Italian seasoning
- ¼ tsp red pepper flakes
- 4 cups spinach
- 2 tbsp fresh lemon juice
- 2 tbsp parsley or chives, minced
- Salt and pepper to taste

DIRECTIONS

1. Follow the instructions on the package to cook the gluten-free pasta. Drain it and toss it with a little olive oil to prevent it from sticking
2. Heat the olive oil and butter in a large saucepan, add the shrimp, and heat through, stirring once until they start to turn pink. Add the Italian seasoning, red pepper flakes, and spinach when the shrimp are almost done. Cook until the spinach has wilted, stirring periodically.
3. Toss the cooked spaghetti with the spinach and shrimp combination. Stir in the remaining butter until it has melted and everything is well combined.
4. Lemon juice, fresh herbs, salt, and pepper to taste. Heat the dish before serving

NUTRITION

- Calories: 368
- Fat: 12 g
- Protein: 5 g
- Carbs: 25 g

Preparation time: 1 hour and 5 minutes
Cooking time: 2 hours
Servings: 1

141. Chocolate Orange Chia Pudding

INGREDIENTS

- 1 cup (240 ml) dairy-free milk
- ¼ cup (40 g) chia seeds
- 3 tbsp cocoa powder
- 1 tsp vanilla extract
- 1 tbsp juice from an orange
- 1 tsp orange zest
- 1–2 tbsp maple syrup

DIRECTIONS

1. Combine all the ingredients in a large jar or bowl. Whisk together until smooth.
2. Refrigerate for at least one hour or overnight after covering
3. Top with orange slices, chocolate chips, extra zest, or anything else you like on top.

NUTRITION

- Calories: 175
- Fat: 1 g
- Protein: 10 g
- Carbs: 21 g

Preparation time: 15 minutes
Cooking time: 10 minutes
Servings: 4

142. Fully Loaded Nachos

INGREDIENTS
- 1 bag of corn chips
- ½ lb taco beef, prepared low-FODMAP
- 1 cup cheddar cheese
- ½ cup Kalamata olives, sliced
- ½ cup lettuce, shredded
- 1 common tomato, diced
- 2 green onions (green parts only), diced
- ¼ cup lactose-free sour cream

DIRECTIONS
1. Preheat the oven to 350°F and line a baking sheet with aluminum foil. Sprinkle ⅓ cheese and ⅓ taco meat over a single layer of chips on the baking sheet. Sprinkle ⅓ of the cheese, ⅓ of the taco meat, and ⅓ of the olives over the second layer of chips. Finish with a final layer of chips with the remaining cheese, meat, and ⅓ of the olives. 5 minutes in the oven (or until the cheese has melted).
2. Remove nachos from the oven and top with the remaining ⅓ of the olives, lettuce, tomatoes, and green onions. For best results, serve sour cream on the side. Warm the dish before serving

NUTRITION
- Calories: 462 kcal
- Fat: 36 g
- Protein: 21 g
- Carbs: 12 g

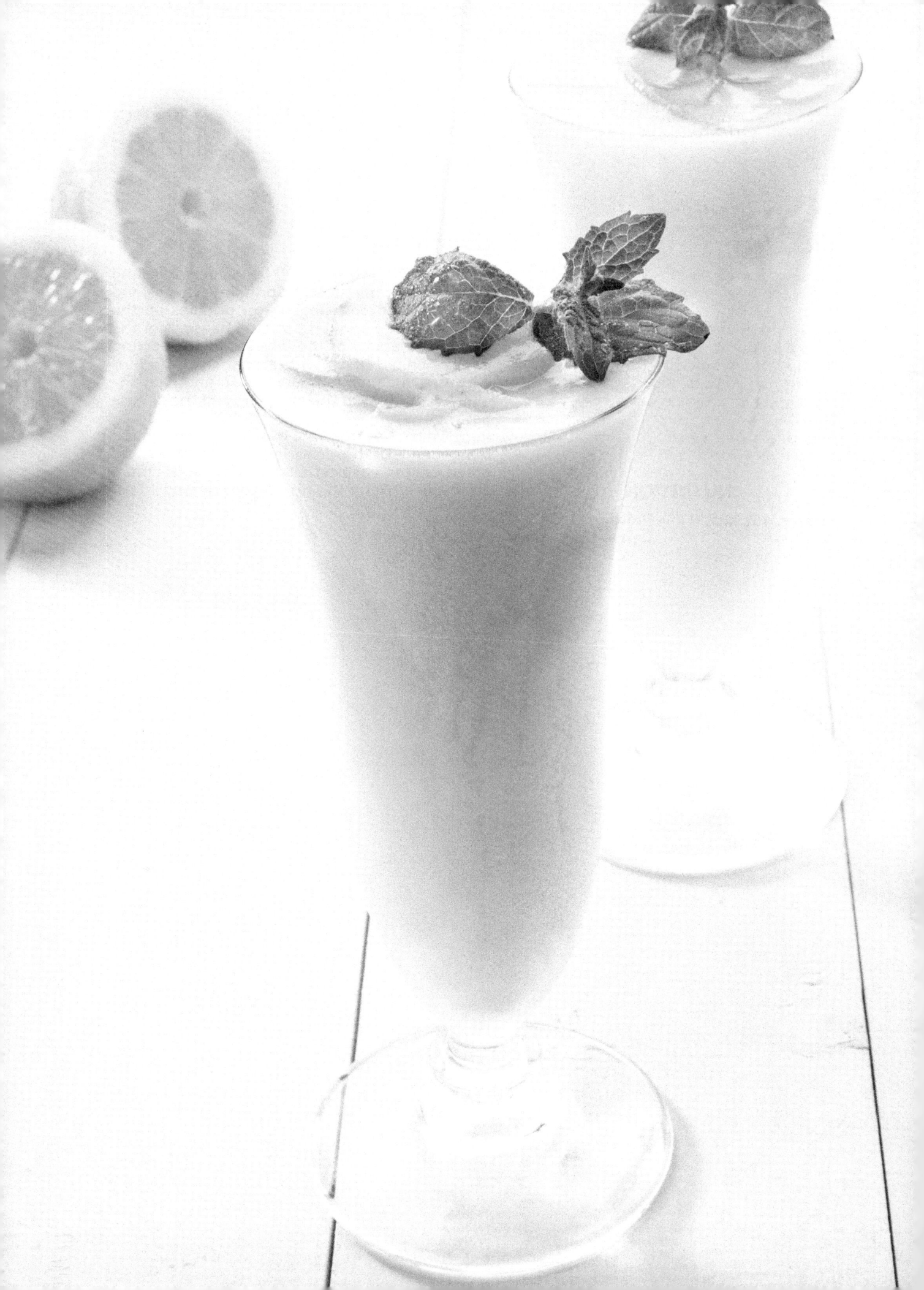

Chapter 15. High-Fiber Recipes

143. Apricot Bars

Preparation time: 5 minutes
Cooking time: 0 minutes
Servings: 2-4

INGREDIENTS
- 1 cup dried apricots
- ½ cup dates pitted
- ½ cup almonds
- ¼ cup coconut

DIRECTIONS
1. In a food processor, add all the ingredients and process until smooth.
2. Line a baking sheet with parchment paper and flatten the mixture into a wide rectangle half a centimeter thick.
3. Before cutting into bars, chill them for at least 30 minutes in the freezer.
4. Refrigerate the bars for up to 1 week or freeze them for 1 month in an airtight container.

NUTRITION
- Calories: 230
- Fat: 17 g
- Protein: 12 g
- Carbs: 46 g

---

144. Spaghetti Squash "Bolognese"

Preparation time: 5 minutes
Cooking time: 0 minutes
Servings: 1

INGREDIENTS
- 1 large spaghetti squash
- 2 cups diced red onion
- 4 garlic cloves, minced
- 2 cups cherry tomatoes
- 1 cup sliced mushrooms (optional)
- 1 tsp chili powder
- 1 tsp poultry seasoning
- 1 tsp garlic powder
- ¼ tsp curry powder
- ¼ tsp sea salt
- ½ cup tomatoes sun-dried
- ¼ cup Brazil nut basil "Parmesan"

For the Brazil nut basil "Parmesan":
- ¼ cup Brazil nuts
- ¼ tsp sea salt
- ¼ tsp dried basil
- 1 garlic clove

DIRECTIONS
1. Preheat the oven to 400°F. With a sharp knife, carefully cut the spaghetti squash in half and remove the seeds. Place the squash halves cut-side down on a baking sheet filled with 12 inches of water. Bake for 30-40 minutes, or until a finger inserted slightly into the squash shell leaves an indentation. Remove the squash halves from the oven and set them aside. When the squash is cool enough to handle, scrape out the inside with a fork to make "spaghetti" strips. The squash noodles should be divided into 2 bowls.
2. To prepare the "Bolognese", combine the chopped onion and water in a medium saucepan. Over medium-high heat, sauté the onion until translucent and soft. To prevent sticking, add water by tablespoonfuls as needed. Cook, stirring regularly, for 5-7 minutes, until the tomatoes soften, add the garlic, cherry tomatoes, mushrooms, chili powder, curry powder, sea salt, poultry seasoning, garlic powder, and sun-dried tomatoes to the pot. Blend the sauce components in an immersion blender until incorporated, but still lumpy. Transfer to a stand mixer and process until smooth, leaving the lid ajar to allow steam to escape. Serve the spaghetti squash with the sauce on top. Enjoy with a spoonful of basil Parmesan with Brazil nuts on top.
3. To prepare the Parmesan, crush the Brazil nuts, basil, sea salt, and garlic until small crumbs form in a blender or food processor.

NUTRITION
- Calories: 117
- Fat: 13 g
- Protein: 10 g
- Carbs: 46 g

Preparation time: 5 minutes
Cooking time: 0 minutes
Servings: 3-4

145. Lemon Sorbet

INGREDIENTS

- ¾ cup honey
- 3 sage leaves
- 1 ½ cups water
- 1 cup lemon juice (from about 6 lemons) fresh-squeezed
- 1 tbsp lemon zest

DIRECTIONS

1. In a small saucepan, combine the sage leaves, honey, and 1 ½ cup of water. Heat over medium heat, stirring constantly, until honey is completely dissolved. Combine lemon zest and juice in a mixing bowl. Refrigerate after stirring well. Remove and discard sage leaves.
2. In an ice cream maker, process the remaining ingredients according to the manufacturer's instructions. If you do not have an ice cream maker, place ingredients in a bowl and freeze for 30 minutes, stirring well every 30 minutes until it reaches the right consistency.

NUTRITION

- Calories: 78
- Fat: 2 g
- Protein: 55 g
- Carbs: 15 g

Preparation time: 5 minutes
Cooking time: 0 minutes
Servings: 2

146. Raspberry and Lime Chia Parfait

INGREDIENTS

- 1 cup fresh or froz en raspberries
- 1 cup unsweetened almond milk
- 2 tbsp maple syrup or raw honey
- 1 tsp lime zest
- 1 tsp lime juice
- 3 tbsp chia seeds

For the toppings:
- ½ banana, thinly sliced
- ¼ cup fresh raspberries
- ¼ cup wild blueberries fresh or defrosted

DIRECTIONS

1. In a bowl, mash the raspberries with a fork until smooth. Combine the almond or coconut milk, maple syrup, raw honey, lime zest and juice, and chia seeds in a large mixing bowl.
2. Let soak for 2-3 hours, or until the mixture is thick and gelatinous. Serve the chia pudding with bananas, raspberries, and blueberries in 2 jars or bowls.

NUTRITION

- Calories: 157
- Fat: 10 g
- Protein: 5 g
- Carbs: 15 g

Preparation time: 5 minutes
Cooking time: 0 minute
Servings: 4

147. Black Bean Hummus Crudité Platter

INGREDIENTS

- ½ cup dried black beans
- ½ cup ripe avocado, peeled and diced
- ¼ cup cilantro leaves
- ½ jalapeño, seeded and roughly chopped
- 4 tbsp lime juice, freshly squeezed
- ½ tbsp finely chopped garlic
- ½ tsp ground cumin
- ½ tsp ground coriander
- Salt and pepper

For the crudités:
- 4–5 orange and purple carrots, peeled and cut into wedges
- 6 radishes, cut into wedges
- 3 small Persian cucumbers, cut into slices and wedges
- 1 yellow bell pepper, cut into wedges
- 1 red bell pepper, cut into wedges
- 3 celery stalks, cut into sticks
- 10 cherry tomatoes

DIRECTIONS

1. Drain and discard the liquid if using dried black beans. Fill a medium saucepan half full with water and set aside. Bring to a boil, then reduce to a simmer and simmer for 45–75 minutes, or until the vegetables are very soft. Drain the beans and reserve 4 tbsp of the cooking liquid.
2. In a food processor or blender, puree the cooked and canned beans, jalapeño, cilantro, lime juice, avocado, garlic, ground cumin, coriander, and reserved cooking water from the can until very smooth. Salt and pepper to taste.
3. Arrange the prepared vegetable crudités on a plate. Fill a bowl halfway with the hummus and top with fresh cilantro. Serve with the crudités.

NUTRITION

- Calories: 313
- Fat: 16 g
- Protein: 13 g
- Carbs: 33 g

Preparation time: 5 minutes
Cooking time: 0 minutes
Servings: 1

148. Celery Juice

INGREDIENTS
- 1 bunch celery

DIRECTIONS
1. Clean the celery by rinsing it and running it through a juicer. Drink it as soon as possible to get the optimal benefits.
2. Alternatively, you can chop the celery and puree it until smooth in a high-powered blender. Strain carefully and consume immediately.

NUTRITION
- Calories: 20
- Fat: 1 g
- Protein: 2 g
- Carbs: 3 g

Preparation time: 5 minutes
Cooking time: 15 minutes
Servings: 1

149. Sweet Potato Chips

INGREDIENTS
- 2 large sweet potatoes
- 2 tsp coconut oil (optional)
- ¼ tsp sea salt
- ¼ tsp garlic powder
- ¼ tsp cumin
- ¼ tsp paprika
- ¼ tsp chili powder
- ⅛ tsp cayenne (optional)

DIRECTIONS
1. Preheat the oven to 250°F. Slice the sweet potatoes very thinly with a mandolin or knife, about ¹⁄₁₆ inch thick if possible and no more than ⅛ inch thick. Make sure they are thin and uniform but not translucent. Bring water to a boil in a saucepan. Return the sweet potato slices to medium heat once they have been added to the boiling water. Remove the sweet potatoes and drain the water after 5 minutes.
2. In a small bowl, combine the sea salt, cumin, paprika, garlic powder, chili powder, poultry seasoning, and cayenne. Lightly grease 2 baking sheets with coconut oil. Lay the sweet potato slices on the trays in a non-overlapping pattern. Brush the tops of the sweet potatoes with a little more coconut oil. Over the top of the slices, sprinkle generously with the spice mixture.
3. Preheat the oven to 350°F and bake the sweet potatoes for 25 minutes. Remove the pans from the oven and set aside any slices that are already crispy. Return the pans to the oven for another 5 minutes and check to see if the crispy slices have been removed. Bake the remaining slices for another 3–5 minutes if necessary. Note that the chips may not appear crispy when initially removed from the oven, but will crisp up as they cool.
4. Serve the sweet potato chips with guacamole or eat them on their own. Within a few hours of creating them, their crispiness is just right.

NUTRITION
- Calories: 150
- Fat: 10 g
- Protein: 2 g
- Carbs: 16 g

Preparation time: 5 minutes
Cooking time: 0 minutes
Servings: 1

150. Guacamole

INGREDIENTS

- 2 avocados
- ½ lemon
- 1 lime
- 1 small tomato, finely diced
- ¼ red onion, finely diced
- ½ cup cilantro, chopped
- 1 garlic clove, minced
- ¼ jalapeño, minced (optional)
- ¼ tsp sea salt (optional)

DIRECTIONS

1. In a small bowl, mash the avocado with lemon or lime juice.
2. Mix the mashed avocado with the tomato, garlic, jalapeño, onion, cilantro, and sea salt.
3. Serve with sweet potato chips, chopped vegetables of your choice, as a salad dressing, or on top of cooked vegetables as preferred.

NUTRITION

- Calories: 60
- Fat: 5 g
- Protein: 10 g
- Carbs: 3 g

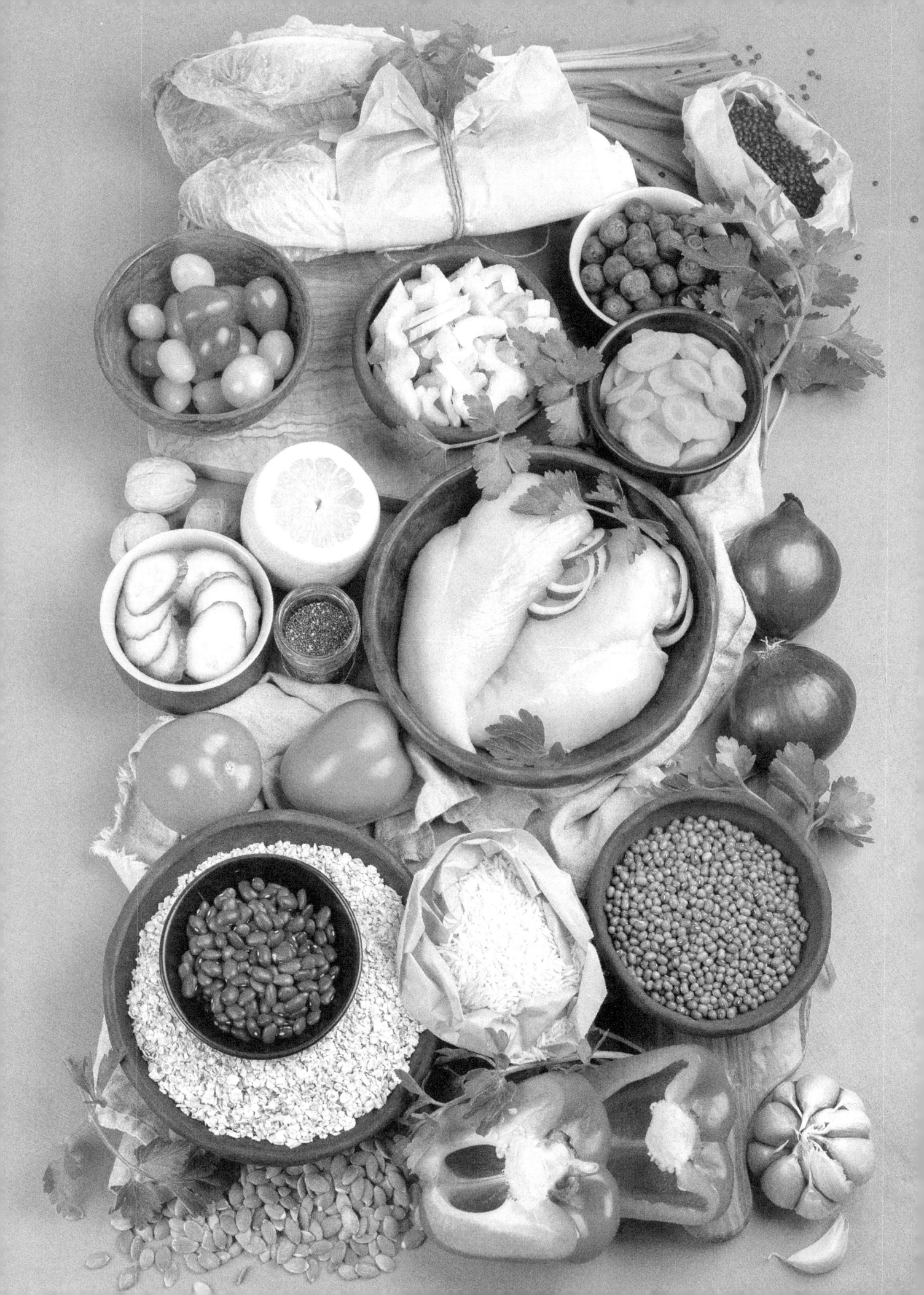

28-Day meal plan

Day	Breakfast	Lunch	Snack	Dinner
1	Fruit Punch	Grilled Vegetable Wrap Recipe With Hummus	Apple and Pistachio Salad on Spinach	Beet Soup
2	Chocolate Pudding	Mediterranean Grilled Chicken Wrap	Apricot Bars	Chicken Burgers
3	Oat Milk	Green Goodness Sandwich	Black Bean Hummus Crudité Platter	Fresh Asparagus Soup
4	Apple Juice	Turkey, Brie, and Apple Sandwich With Apple Cider Mayo	Catalan Style Spinach	Pumpkin Waffles
5	Black Tea	Black Beans and Cauliflower Rice (Gluten-Free, Vegan/Plant-Based)	Celery Juice	Bean Soup
6	Cranberry Juice	Avocado Sauce Pasta	Chocolate Orange Chia Pudding	Carrot Cucumber Salad
7	Banana Almond Milk Smoothie	Greek Quinoa Bowls	Cranberry Almond Oatmeal	Lemon Chicken and Rice
8	Mixed Berry Smoothie	Baked Sweet Potato Tacos	Eggplant Paste	Peachy Pork With Rice
9	Green Smoothie	Sweet Potato Black Bean Chili	Fiber Bars	Loaded Pumpkin Chowder

Day	Breakfast	Lunch	Snack	Dinner
10	Applesauce	Whole-Wheat Pasta With Fresh Tomatoes and Herbs	Fully Loaded Nachos	Creamy Carrot Soup
11	Greek Inspired Cucumber Salad	Honey Mustard Salmon With Shaved Brussel Sprout Salad	Guacamole	Fish Stew
12	Light Veggie Salad	5-Minute Tomato Salad Lentil	Hummus With Tahini and Turmeric	Mushroom Soup
13	Eastern European Soup	Veggies and Apple With Orange Sauce	Lemon Sorbet	Chicken Soup
14	Citrus Glazed Carrots	Cauliflower Rice with Prawns and Veggies	Low-FODMAP French Oven Beef Stew	Pumpkin Casserole
15	Spring Flavored Pasta	Lentils With Tomatoes and Turmeric	Quick Banana Bread Oatmeal	Fresh Tomato Juice
16	Gluten-Free Curry	Fried Rice With Kale	Raspberry and Lime Chia Parfait	Ground Beef Tostada
17	Garden Veggies Quiche	Stir-Fry Tofu and Red Pepper	Roasted Carrot Sticks in a Honey Garlic Marinade	Beef Barley Soup
18	Fluffy Pumpkin Pancakes	Sweet Potato and Bell Pepper Hash With a Fried Egg	Spaghetti Squash "Bolognese"	Ground Beef and Rice Bowls
19	Sper-Tasty Chicken Muffins	5-Ingredient Sweet Potato Black Bean Chili	Spicy Lemon Pasta With Shrimp	Grilled Vegetable Quesadilla

Day	Breakfast	Lunch	Snack	Dinner
20	Classic Zucchini Bread	Quinoa Florentine	Sweet Potato Aioli	Grilled Veggie Sandwich
21	Pineapple Raspberry Parfaits	Tomato Asparagus Frittata	Sweet Potato Chips	Lentil Linguine Stew
22	Berry Chia Pudding	Shrimp and Mango Salsa Lettuce Wraps	Thai Coconut Lime Soup	Lentil Risotto
23	Spinach Avocado Smoothie	Bacon-Wrapped Asparagus	Tomato Cashew Pesto	Lentil Stew
24	Strawberry Pineapple Smoothie	Zucchini Pasta With Shrimp	Veggie-Packed Low-FODMAP Soup	Pasta With Beans and Turkey
25	Peach Blueberry Parfaits	Sweet Potato Buns Sandwich	Apple and Pistachio Salad on Spinach	Pasta With Chicken and Olives
26	Raspberry Yogurt Cereal Bowl	Shrimp, Sausage, and Veggie Skillet	Apricot Bars	Pasta With Spinach and White Beans
27	Avocado Toast	Sea Scallops With Spinach and Bacon	Black Bean Hummus Crudité Platter	Chicken Florentine
28	Loaded Pita Pockets	Liver With Onion and Parsley One	Catalan Style Spinach	Chipotle Black Bean Chili

Goodbye Bye

Conclusion

Without the risk of diverticulitis, you can eat whatever you want. So go ahead and enjoy! However, be sure to exercise often and work out your digestive system by eating lots of fiber-rich foods.

If you have been following this diet from the beginning, then congratulations on making it this far! I really hope you found a way to overcome your condition faster than the average week or two. It takes time for bacteria in our gut to become resistant to what we are doing so be patient; allow time for your body's immune system to get accustomed to new foods.

Once you feel at ease with this diet, then you have the option to start adding some of your older favorites back into your system. I recommend trying a food out for at least a week before throwing it out there again. Because trust me, you do not want to be doing that yo-yo dieting thing!

The last step is maintaining. It's essential to keep eating all of these new foods daily until something else changes in your body that demands making changes. Please remember that no matter what, your problem could come back if you stop caring for yourself and allowing yourself to heal.

I would recommend finding a diet that works best for you, but with the dietary recommendations of this Diverticulitis Diet, I hope you will have the strength to overcome your condition before it becomes severe. This way, even if it does happen to come back, at least you will have learned how to successfully fight it before that happens.

If you have any questions or suggestions that could improve this article, feel free to leave them in the comments section below. Thanks!

Made in United States
North Haven, CT
26 January 2023